Essential Procedures for Practitioners in Emergency, Urgent, and Primary Care Settings

A Clinical Companion

Theresa M. Campo, DNP, APRN, NP-C, received a Doctor of Nursing Practice from Case Western Reserve University in Cleveland, OH, and a Master of Science in Nursing from Widener University in Chester, PA. She has more than 16 years experience in emergency medicine as a Registered Professional Nurse and Advanced Practice Nurse. She is board-certified by the American Academy of Nurse Practitioners as a Family Nurse Practitioner. Currently, she works as a nurse practitioner in the Quick Care Center of the Emergency Department at Shore Memorial Hospital in Southern New Jersey. She is owner and primary lecturer of Farfalla Education, LLC. She is an adjunct professor at Case Western Reserve University and The Richard Stockton College of New Jersey. She has lectured nationally and internationally, as well as authored articles in peer-reviewed journals. She is the column editor of Cases of Note column for the *Advanced Emergency Nursing Journal*.

Keith A. Lafferty, MD, received his BA in Biology cum laude from Holy Family University in 1989 and his MD from the Medical College of Pennsylvania in 1994. At the completion of his training, he was honored by his colleagues who voted him the best senior resident teacher. Following his residency in emergency medicine and a critical care fellowship, he spent 6 years in full academics as a medical student and a critical care director. Dr. Lafferty is currently the Student Clerkship Director at Gulf Coast Medical Center and is an adjunct assistant professor of emergency medicine at Temple University.

As a physician, Dr. Lafferty focuses on the critical care of emergency medicine and practices in both Philadelphia and Florida. As an author, he has written numerous chapters and manuscripts, mostly having to do with critical care procedures of emergency medicine, with an emphasis on the airway. He has presented many of his research papers at local and national levels.

Dr. Lafferty has recently traveled to Haiti, participating in mission expeditions after its devastating earthquake. Those experiences are reminiscent of his own humbled beginnings, growing up with his mother and sister in a Philadelphia housing project. Providing medical care for the most indigent and teaching evidence-based medicine are the essence of his vocation.

Essential Procedures for Practitioners in Emergency, Urgent, and Primary Care Settings

A Clinical Companion

Theresa M. Campo, DNP, APRN, NP-C

Keith A. Lafferty, MD

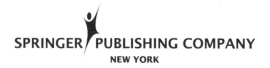

SPRINGER PUBLISHING COMPANY
NEW YORK

Springer Publishing Company, LLC
11 West 42nd Street
New York, NY 10036
www.springerpub.com

Acquisitions Editor: Margaret Zuccarini
Cover Design: David Levy
Composition: Newgen

ISBN: 978-0-8261-1878-3
E-book ISBN: 978-0-8261-1879-0

13/ 5

The author and the publisher of this Work have made every effort to use sources believed to be reliable to provide information that is accurate and compatible with the standards generally accepted at the time of publication. Because medical science is continually advancing, our knowledge base continues to expand. Therefore, as new information becomes available, changes in procedures become necessary. We recommend that the reader always consult current research and specific institutional policies before performing any clinical procedure. The author and publisher shall not be liable for any special, consequential, or exemplary damages resulting, in whole or in part, from the readers' use of, or reliance on, the information contained in this book. The publisher has no responsibility for the persistence or accuracy of URLs for external or third-party Internet Web sites referred to in this publication and does not guarantee that any content on such Web sites is, or will remain, accurate or appropriate.

Library of Congress Cataloging-in-Publication Data

Campo, Theresa M.
   Essential procedures for practitioners in office, urgent, and emergency care settings / Theresa M. Campo, Keith Lafferty.
      p. ; cm.
   Includes bibliographical references and index.
   ISBN 978-0-8261-1878-3 — ISBN 978-0-8261-1879-0 (e-book ISBN)
1. Nurse practitioners–Handbooks, manuals, etc. 2. Physicians' assistants—Handbooks, manuals, etc. 3. Medical protocols–Handbooks, manuals, etc.   I. Lafferty, Keith.   II. Title.
   [DNLM: 1. Wounds and Injuries—therapy—Handbooks. 2. Ambulatory Care—methods—Handbooks.
3. Anesthesia—methods—Handbooks. 4. Emergency Medical Services—methods—Handbooks. 5. Nurse Practitioners—Handbooks. 6. Physician Assistants—Handbooks.   WO 39 C198e 2010]
   RT82.8.C36 2010
   610.73092—dc22   2010025697

Special discounts on bulk quantities of our books are available to corporations, professional associations, pharmaceutical companies, health care organizations, and other qualifying groups.

If you are interested in a custom book, including chapters from more than one of our titles, we can provide that service as well.

For details, please contact:
Special Sales Department
Springer Publishing Company, LLC
11 West 42nd Street, 15th Floor
New York, NY 10036-8002
Phone: 877-687-7476 or 212-431-4370
Fax: 212-941-7842
E-mail: sales@springerpub.com

Printed in the United States of America by Bang Printing.

*This book evolved from the experiences and encounters I have had
with mentors, students, colleagues, and patients who have not only
aided in the development of my career but also have influenced my
life. Clinical experiences alone do not make a person grow;
the people along the journey do.*

*Mom, you always said your children were the wind beneath your
wings and now I am riding the wind of your angelic wings.*

*This book is dedicated to my husband, Jonathan Campo. You are my
best friend and soul mate. Thank you for always standing by me with
encouragement, pride, and most of all, love. You have put up with
early mornings, late nights, and just plain long days in completing this
book, yet you never complained. Your words are always of support and
pride and I greatly appreciate them and you. You are the love of my
life and you complete me. Everything I do is because of you. I love you!*

Theresa M. Campo, DNP

*At every one of my encounters with patients, I know my actions are
guided by the thoughts, principles, and passions of my mentors:
Dr. Lynda Micikas, Dr. Robert McNamara, and Dr. David Wagner.
It is not only an honor to have been trained by the "best of the best,"
but even more so to be a disciple of these pioneers and their
relentless cause for perfection. I only hope the students I'm
privileged to teach are able to sense the illumination passed down
to me, in order that they may also attempt to make this
greatest of arts into the greatest science possible.*

*The time, commitment, and dedication creating this manuscript are
small in comparison to the sacrifice given by my beautiful family.
Cathy, you are my love and my soul mate. I am a truly a better person
because of you, and I love you more every day.
Karli, Koko, and Kory, daddy loves you so much.*

Keith A. Lafferty, MD

Contents

IV. SKIN AND WOUND MANAGEMENT PROCEDURES

V. PROCEDURES FOR THE MANAGEMENT OF NAIL AND NAILBED INJURIES

VI. INCISION AND DRAINAGE PROCEDURES

VII. PROCEDURES FOR EXAMINATION AND TREATMENT OF COMMON EYE INJURIES

VIII. PROCEDURES FOR MANAGING COMMON NOSE CONDITIONS

IX. PROCEDURES FOR MANAGING COMMON EAR INJURIES

X. PROCEDURES FOR EXAMINATION AND MANAGEMENT OF COMMON DENTAL INJURIES

XI. PROCEDURES FOR MANAGING COMMON MUSCULOSKELETAL CONDITIONS AND INJURIES

XII. PROCEDURES FOR MANAGING COMMON GASTROINTESTINAL CONDITIONS

XIII. PROCEDURES FOR MANAGING COMMON GENITOURINARY CONDITIONS

XIV. PROCEDURES FOR PERFORMING SKIN BIOPSY

Contributors

Lee Ann Boyd, MSN, ARNP-C, CUNP
Southwest Florida Urologic Associates, Cape Coral, Florida

Joseph Hong, MD
Atlantic Dermatology and Laser Center, Linwood, New Jersey

Larry Isaacs, MD, FACEP, FAAEM
Director, Emergency Department, Virtua Hospital, Voorhees Division,
Voorhees, New Jersey

Photography

Cathy Lafferty
Cape May, New Jersey

Joseph McDonough
Petersburg, New Jersey

Reviewers

David Angelastro, MD, FACEP
Director Emergency Medicine, Bayfront Emergency Physicians, Shore Memorial Hospital, Somers Point, New Jersey

Omar Benitez, MD
Southwest Floridaorida Urologic Associates, Cape Coral, Florida

Anne Marie Burkhardt, MSN, FNPC
Emergency Physician Associates, Atlanticare Regional Medical Center, Atlantic City, New Jersey

Teresa Byrd, MSN, NP-C
Ocean City Family Practice, Ocean City, New Jersey

James Cancilleri, DPM, FACFAS, FAPWCA
Private Podiatric Practice, Somers Point, New Jersey

Debra D. Fett Desmond, MD
Staff Physician/Owner, Dermatology Solutions, Fort Myers, Florida

Valerie Dyke, MD
The Colorectal Institute, Fort Myers, Florida

Victor Robert Frankel, MD
The Frankel Orthopedic and Sports Medicine Center, LLC, Linwood, New Jersey

Richard Juda, MD
Department of Critical Care, Gulf Coast Hospital, Fort Myers, Florida

Charles H. Nolte, DO
Team Health East Emergency Physician, Virtua Health System, Voorhees, New Jersey

William Schumacher, DO, FACEP
Bayfront Emergency Physicians, Shore Memorial Hospital, Somers Point, New Jersey

Craig Stafford, DMD, PC
Private Practice—General Dentistry, Lancaster, Pennsylvania

Foreword

As the title suggests, *Essential Procedures for Practitioners in Emergency, Urgent, and Primary Care Settings* is a book of procedures for practitioners to use in emergency, urgent, and primary care settings. This distinctive book will assist providers in performing procedures commonly done in these settings. This user-friendly, easy to understand, procedurally focused resource offers the necessary background information, illustrations, and step-by-step instructions for providing safe and efficient treatment to patients in these care settings not only the novice, but for experts in emergent and urgent care.

The goal of *Essential Procedures for Practitioners in Emergency, Urgent, and Primary Care Settings* is to provide today's providers with the most up-to-date information available in a concise and systematic framework. Procedures are those that providers see on a daily basis. Theresa M. Campo, DNP, APRN, NP-C and Keith A. Lafferty, MD, coauthors and coeditors, offer a wealth of information and knowledge. This, combined with the expertise of Springer Publishing, ensures you will want to add this book, not only to your medical library collection but also in your clinical setting.

This is the first edition of this book. As practice evolves, new knowledge is acquired and procedures may change. In the meantime, we know you will enjoy utilizing *Essential Procedures for Practitioners in the Emergency, Urgent, and Primary Care Settings*.

K. Sue Hoyt, PhD, RN, FNP-BC, CEN, FAEN, FAANP
Emergency Nurse Practitioner
St. Mary Medical Center
Long Beach, California
Hoyt and Associates, Education and Consultation
San Diego, California

Elda G. Ramirez, PhD, RN, FNP-BC, FAANP
Associate Professor Clinical Nursing
Director of Simulation and Clinical Performance Lab
    and Emergency Concentration
University of Texas Health Science Center Houston
Houston, Texas

Preface

Welcome to the only book of procedures for practitioners in emergency, urgent, and primary care settings. The intention of this book is to aid the practitioner (advanced practice nurse and physician assistant) and student in performing common procedures in these settings. It is meant to be a clinical companion that is easy to understand and follow.

This book has been prepared by clinical experts with numerous years of experience in both academic and clinical arenas of their respective fields. Using the most up-to-date literature as well as experience-based pearls of practice, we have organized this book to be user friendly and broad-based. As busy clinicians, we all understand the time constraints and need for a well-organized and simplified procedural book.

The book is divided into 14 units covering the spectrum of common procedures performed by practitioners in the emergency, urgent, and primary care settings. This collection of thoroughly described procedures is intended for use as a clinical companion and is an easy-to-use reference when performing such techniques. Current evidence-based literature has been used during the writing of this book. For ease of reading, all references are noted at the end of each chapter.

Chapters are organized in a format describing the background, including pathophysiology, of particular disorders requiring the procedure to be performed. Current treatments along with the actual procedures are outlined in each chapter. It is the intent of the authors to purposely describe in some detail the disease process for a better understanding of the indication and performance of the procedure.

Classroom didactic accompanied with hands-on experience are recommended by the authors before performing any procedures. Practitioners should always work within the scope of practice designated by their practicing bodies in their respective states and institutions. The authors and contributors are not responsible for any actions resulting from the use of this text.

Anyone is entitled to their own opinions but not to their own facts. The authors of this book strongly believe that evidence-based practice is the only way to effectively treat patients.

Theresa M. Campo
Keith A. Lafferty

1

The Basics of Patient Procedures: Universal Precautions, Infection Control, Patient Preparation, and Education

Theresa M. Campo

INTRODUCTION

Universal precautions and infection control are keys to minimizing the spread of infection to the health care workers, patients, and family members. In our age of resistance, it is becoming more challenging to effectively treat bacterial infections. Consistent practices of hand hygiene and universal precautions can be the best defense against infections such as methicillin-resistant *Staphylococcus aureus* (MRSA) and other nosocomial infections.

Proper patient preparation and education are methods of ensuring time efficiency when performing procedures and of increasing a patient's level of satisfaction with the health care system. This book will illustrate how to effectively prepare for each procedure in a confident, organized, and time-efficient manner. It will also cover important educational points to share with patients to ensure a rapid and complete recovery.

UNIVERSAL PRECAUTIONS

Universal precautions, sometimes referred to as standard precautions, have been practiced since the late 1980s when the Centers for Disease Control (CDC) published guidelines recommended for use by all health care workers to protect themselves from contamination from body fluids. Universal precautions are defined as "An approach to infection control in which all human blood, tissue, and certain fluids are treated as if known to be infectious for HIV, HBV, and other blood-borne pathogens" (Stedman, 2008). The CDC recommendations should be followed when the risk of contact with any body fluids and/or secretions is present or suspected. These precautions replaced the traditional isolation category of blood and body fluids precautions.

Universal precautions apply not only to visible blood and body fluids, but also to nonvisible semen, vaginal fluids, tissue, and other fluids (e.g., amniotic, cerebrospinal, pleural, peritoneal, etc.). Other bodily excretions and secretions do not require universal precautions unless blood is visualized or suspected. Examples include feces, nasal secretions, sputum, sweat, tears, urine, and vomitus (cdc.gov, 2010).

Implementing universal precautions includes using barriers to protect the health care worker from contamination. Examples of these protective barriers include gloves, masks, goggles, and gowns. Additional precautions must be taken to protect health care workers from needle puncture by using needleless systems and needle-free products, and the use of vacutainers when possible. The required degree of protection depends upon the potential threat to the health care worker for exposure to infected bodily fluids.

Gloves should be worn whenever the potential for contact with blood or body fluids arises. They should also be worn if handling contaminated items such as sheets, absorbent pads, bedside tables, and other equipment. Gloves should be changed if their integrity is compromised (ripped, punctured, or torn) after patient contact and if grossly contaminated. Hand washing should always be performed before and after wearing gloves.

Masks, protective eyewear, and gowns should be utilized during any patient contact or procedure where the risk of contact with fluids and/or tissue is present. These barrier methods are best worn if splashing of the fluid is a potential threat, for example, droplets of blood or fluids, mucous membrane droplets (sneezing, coughing, etc.), or splashing of blood or body fluids during a procedure (active bleeding from a vein or artery, fluid under extreme pressure such as the contents of an abscess).

INFECTION CONTROL

Infection control procedures are important in protecting both the health care worker and the patient. In addition to using the universal precautions, basic hand washing is key in preventing the spread of infection to the health care worker as well as to other patients. Hand washing before and after any patient contact, with or without gloves, should be part of everyday practice. Hand washing has reduced the rate of nosocomial infections and MRSA transmission (Barnes & Jinks, 2009). Creamer et al. (2010) demonstrated that MRSA was present on the finger tips of health care workers ($n = 523$) even after hand hygiene practices with either 4% alcohol, chlorhexidine, or soap and water. They also found MRSA present on the finger tips of health care workers who had contact with the patient, the patient's environment, and even with no specific contact (Creamer et al., 2010).

Debate continues whether hand washing is the sole method of cleansing the hands. Alcohol-based hand sanitizers are an alternative and accepted method of proper hand cleansing. The current recommendations state that hand rubbing with an approved sanitizer can be more effective than hand washing with soap and water. This method is best when cleansing between patients, with hand washing being the best method for gross contamination. Hand washing should be done for a minimum of 15 seconds to be effective.

Good hand washing techniques and universal precautions are to be implemented before and after all procedures presented in this book. Gloves, gowns, and protective eye wear should be worn whenever there is potential exposure to blood or body fluids. Use of needleless or needle-free products is encouraged but is dependent on what equipment your institution provides.

PATIENT PREPARATION

Preparing the patient, mentally and physically, for a procedure is as important as performing the procedure. All procedures, whether seemingly basic and trivial or obviously more advanced and emergent, are invasive to the patient and should be discussed with the patient in as much detail as the situation allows. Discussions should include the potential risks and benefits of performing the procedure versus not performing the procedure and should include the required follow-up and care. Care should be taken to include options if various techniques are available for the particular situation at hand (i.e., suture closure versus skin adhesive) and the risks and benefits of each method.

Continued reassurance should be given not only to the patient but also to the family member(s). Communicating confidence to the patient and family member(s) during the initial discussion makes a difference in the course of the procedure. When speaking to a patient, remember to keep your voice low and slow, and to pause at regular intervals to provide the patient the opportunity to ask questions. Always speak directly to the patient, even if the patient is a young child. You may need to first calm and reassure the parent before you can proceed to explain a procedure to the pediatric patient. Upon completion of the discussion, allow ample time for questions and further discussions. After explaining the intended procedure, consent must be obtained before initiating the procedure. Confidence and trust go a long way. Remember, anxiety spreads faster than fire.

Every effort should be made to make the patient and family member comfortable for the procedure. Place the patient in a comfortable position, especially if the procedure will be lengthy. Have the family member sit in a secure chair on the opposite side of the stretcher/examination table, so he or she is not only out of the way but in case the family member becomes "squeamish." Have your assistant also stand on the opposite side so that he or she can not only assist you but also ensure the visitor remains safe during the procedure.

In this book, the required equipment is listed in the "Procedural Preparation" section of the chapters. All efforts to list what will be needed as well as alternative equipment have been made. Developing a checklist of equipment is helpful for the provider and his/her assistant to ensure everything that is needed will be at the bedside. Exiting to obtain necessary equipment during the procedure is time consuming and may have a negative effect on the patient's confidence.

Once the equipment is at the bedside and consent has been obtained, continued reassurance should be given to the patient and any family members present. Parents and family members should be allowed at the bedside when appropriate; this should be up to the provider's discretion. Universal precautions should be strictly followed for procedures involving or potentially involving blood and body fluid. When performing the procedure, every effort should be made to be in a comfortable position. Body mechanics are key for the provider as well as the assistants. Some procedures can be lengthy and stress the neck and back. Simple measures to ensure proper body mechanics and comfortable positioning are sitting in a chair, adjusting the height of the stretcher/examination table, having the patient positioned close to you to avoid reaching, and maintaining proper lighting.

PATIENT EDUCATION

Taking the time to properly educate the patient on follow-up, medications, wound care, and so on can save time and frustration to the patient and provider. Verbal instructions followed by written instructions are the ideal situation. Taking the time to review the procedure that was performed, proper care and management at home, and follow-up are key components of any discharge instructions. Always allow time for questions and further discussion to ensure the patient and family member have a good understanding.

Patient's anxiety levels, medications, and even simply the trauma of experiencing a procedure can effect what information the patient actually absorbs. Providing written instructions assists the patient and guides his/her follow-up. Written instructions can be obtained through software companies specializing in patient instructions or via the Internet. Always fully review the instructions before distributing to your patients. Instructions that are consistently updated based on current evidence-based practice are best. Review and update of the instructions for accuracy and current measures should be done on a daily basis.

Whenever instructions are given to a patient, ample time, should again, be given for review and questions. It can be frustrating for a patient with questions to be rushed out of the examination area. The patient either returns upset and angry or continuously calls to clarify the instructions. Such patients may never return for follow-up or continued care.

Documentation of verbal and written instruction is extremely important. Be sure to document what was discussed and provided to the patient, the place and time for follow-up (i.e., PCP, ED, urgent care, or specialist), whether the patient and/or family member verbalized understanding of the instructions and specific questions that were addressed. Detail is key.

SUMMARY

Take a time-out break before starting any procedure. Review the particular procedure in this book and then review it once again in your head. Plan how to proceed and envision the parameters of the procedures before you begin. Take a deep breath. Doing this will help to ensure that you place yourself in a comfortable position that will sustain you throughout the procedure. There is nothing worse than bending over too far or standing during a time-consuming procedure and suffering a resultant stiff back or sore legs. When possible, sit on an adjustable chair or stool while performing a procedure. Adjustments can be made during the procedure, if necessary, to avoid bending over for prolonged periods of time causing posture strain that can lead to provider discomfort, pain, sloppiness, and inferior results. Be sure to take care of yourself before taking care of others.

Universal precautions, and patient preparation and education are key elements to any procedure performed in the emergency, urgent, or primary care setting. Providers need to deliver high quality, efficient care while keeping the patient comfortable and calm. Achieving these goals requires extra steps to prepare properly for the procedure, to educate your patient and family, and to be compassionate during every patient encounter. It is always important to treat your patients as if they were your family or close friend.

RESOURCES

Barnes, T. A., & Jinks, A. (2009). Methicillin resistant *Staphylococcus aureus*: The modern-day challenge. *British Journal of Nursing, 27*, 14–18.

Creamer, E., Dorrian, S., Dolan, A., Sherlock, O., Fitzgerald-Hughes, D., Thomas, T., et al. (2010). When are the hands of health care workers positive for methicillin resistant *Staphylococcus aureus? The Journal of Hospital Infection, 75*(2), 107–111.

Croft, A. C., & Woods, G. L. (2007). Specimen collection and handling for diagnosis of infectious disease. In R. A. McPherson & M. R. Pincus (Eds.), *Henry's clinical diagnosis and management by laboratory methods* (21st ed.) Retrieved from http://www.mdconsult.com/das/book/body/187068169–3/962478166/1393/484.html#4-u1.0-B1-4160-0287-1..50067-7-cesec8_4418

Del Rio, C. (2008). Prevention of human immunodeficiency virus infection. In L. Goldman & D. A. Ausiello (Eds.), *Cecil's medicine* (23rd ed.). Retrieved from http://www.mdconsult.com/das/book/body/187068169–3/962478166/1492/1372.html#4-u1.0-B978-1-4160-2805-5..50416-X–cesec15_17320

Henderson, D. K. (2010). Immunodeficiency virus in health care settings. In G. L. Mandell, J. E. Bennett, & R. Dolin (Eds.), *Principles and practice of infectious diseases* (7th ed.). Retrieved from http://www.mdconsult.com/book/player/book.do?method=display&type=bookPage&decorator=header&eid=4-u1.0-B978-0-443-06839-3..00306-4-s0080&displayedEid=4-u1.0-B978-0-443-06839-3..00306-4-s0085&uniq=187068169&isbn=978-0-443-06839-3&sid=962478166

Lafferty, K. (2006). Femoral phlebotomy: The vacuum tube method is preferable over needle syringe. *Journal of Emergency Medicine, 31*(1), 83–85.

Lederer, J. W. (2009). A comprehensive hand washing approach to reducing MRSA health care associated infections. *Joint Commission Journal of Quality and Patient Safety, 35*(4), 180–185.

Messina, M. J., Brodell, L.A., & Brodell, R.T. (2008). Hand hygiene in the dermatologist office: To wash or to rub? *Journal of the American Academy of Dermatology, 59*(6), 1043–1049.

Nicholau, D., & Arnold, W. P. (2010). Environmental safety including chemical dependency. In R. D. Miller (Ed.), *Miller's anesthesia* (7th ed.). Retrieved from http://www.mdconsult.com/das/book/body/187068169-3/962478166/2053/104.html#4-u1.0-B978-0-443-06959-8..00101-1–s0210_6196

Stedman (2008). *Stedman's concise medical dictionary for the health professions and nursing* (6th ed). Philadelphia, PA: Wolters Kluwer Health.

2

Consent

THERESA M. CAMPO

INTRODUCTION

The legal aspects of medicine and nursing are often overlooked and yet are very important. Obtaining the proper consent, becoming familiar with the ethics of good practice, documenting thoroughly and accurately, and learning about insurance reimbursement are integral aspects of practicing medicine and performing procedures. Having even a basic understanding can aid the provider in making good, sound decisions for the patient, health care team, and self.

CONSENT

Consent can be defined as "to give approval, assent, or permission. A person must be of sufficient mental capacity and of the age at which he or she is legally recognized as competent to give consent (age of consent)" (http://medical-dictionary.thefreedictionary.com/consent). Informed consent is the patient's right to be presented with sufficient information about a recommended procedure by the provider or a representative for the purpose of enabling the patient to make an informed decision. Patients or their representatives have the right to fully participate in this decision. As the health care professional recommending the procedure, the senior health care provider must participate in the process of explaining the procedure or treatment being offered to the patient, including the risks, benefits, and alternatives. In certain situations, a student can explain the procedure to the patient along with the relevant benefits and risks, as long as the student is accompanied by the health care professional who is responsible for the patient. The essential elements that must be presented to the patient include: diagnosis, the purpose of the treatment or procedure, what the procedure entails, the possible risks/benefits, the alternative risks of not receiving the treatment or procedure, prognosis, and consequences if the treatment is not provided at all. Patients must be deemed competent in order to sign or verbalize consent.

Informed or "understood" consent is necessary for any patient who is physically touched and for any invasive procedure. Not obtaining this beforehand can lead to communication discrepancies. Informed consent can be divided into two areas: expressed consent and implied consent. All forms of consent have become more important due to the increasing amount of litigation in the health care field.

Expressed consent is where the patient consents to treatment or procedures through direct words. This can be written or verbal. *Written consent* requirements are stipulated by individual hospitals and mandated by the Joint Commission. Written consent is used as a method of proof that the information was explained to the patient/patient representative and is valid for 30 days. Verbal consent can be obtained and then documented on the chart, but requires two witnesses to verify the consent. *Implied consent* can be obtained through the patient's behavior. One example of implied consent is when patients wait for hours to get the H1N1 influenza vaccine.

Emergency consent can be obtained when there is risk to the patient's life or if serious impairment to life or limb can occur with no intervention. The provider may act with responsibility to avert loss of limb or life. Examples of this include cardiac arrest, trauma, and significant fracture with neurovascular compromise. However, a patient's relatives or members of the health care team cannot give consent on behalf of patients who are incompetent or unconscious in a non-emergent situation unless they possess power of attorney status (Jawaid & Jawaid, 2006).

Consent for minors must be obtained from either their parent or legal guardian. A family representative can give consent for treatment as long as it is in writing from the parent or guardian. Minors may be treated as adults if they are emancipated (legally free of parental control). Emancipation can occur by being a mature minor, married, being parents themselves, or being in active military service. In some states a 14 or 15 year old may be considered a mature minor and, therefore, may give consent for their own care. Reference your individual state laws regarding minors as they vary for each state. However, although the child cannot give consent for the procedure, the procedure should be explained in terms that the child will understand.

Anyone who is competent, autonomous, and not experiencing central nervous system dysfunction (i.e. alcohol, drugs, ischemia, or metabolic derangement) has the right to refuse treatment even if the provider feels it is necessary. Make sure that the patient is aware of any risks for not having the procedure or treatment. Always refer to your institution's policy and procedures with regard to consent as they differ from institution to institution, and state to state.

Prior to beginning any procedure discussed in this book, discuss the procedure, potential complications, risks, benefits, and alternatives with the patient. In addition, discuss the importance of follow-up and the expected time to return to the treatment area or primary care provider for reevaluation. Consent should be obtained based on your institution's policies and procedures.

OTHER LEGAL CONSIDERATIONS

Malpractice is a concern for providers with regard to health care delivery, especially when performing procedures. Malpractice is defined as when the provider deviates from the standard of practice through an act or omission that can result in injury or complication to the patient. Providers must be cognizant of the most current guidelines and standards of practice. Care must be taken to "first do no harm," which can be accomplished by regular review of the current literature, regulations, and practice guidelines.

Ethical issues can also lead to legal ramifications. Cultural, ethnic, and religious beliefs can place the provider in a difficult situation. What is standard care for the majority of the patient population may not be acceptable to the patient based on one or many of these factors. Receiving blood products or certain medications and treatments may be thought to be detrimental or unacceptable by a particular religious group, culture, or ethnic group. When the provider faces this situation, he or she should always consult the ethics committee of their institution immediately whether the outcome of altered or no treatment can be potentially life threatening. It is often very difficult for providers to "sit and wait" for an acceptable conclusion.

Respecting the patient's beliefs and practices can be frustrating and difficult. However, it may be a priority of the patient, not necessarily the provider. Always engage a collaborative approach with the patient, family, community, and health care team.

Medical liability and resulting litigation are a great concern for every provider. Medical malpractice reform, tort reform, and capitation are methods to better regulate this rapidly growing problem. The medical record has become more of a weapon in the provider's defense of lawsuits and litigation. Proper and thorough documentation are essential for not only preventing litigation, but also positively effecting reimbursement from third-party payers.

DOCUMENTATION AND REIMBURSEMENT

The medical document creates and reflects pertinent information with regard to history, physical examination, plan of care (episodic and/or continual), and diagnosis. Communication paired with thorough documentation can promote realistic expectations for the patient and help protect the provider against malpractice allegations. Documentation needs to be complete and legible for claims review, quality management, and peer review.

The Centers for Medicare and Medicaid (CMS) have published evaluation and management (E&M) guidelines for physician and health care provider documentation. The medical encounter must include seven components for defining the level of service provided. They are:

1. History*
   - History of presenting illness (HPI)
   - Review of systems (ROS)
   - Past family, surgical history (PFSH)
   - Type of history
2. Exam*
3. Medical decision making*
4. Counseling
5. Coordination of care
6. Nature of presenting problem
7. Time

Documentation and determination of the level of billable care provided are charged as one of five levels of complexity. They are described by the nature of the

---

*Key components.

decision making, the extent of the history, the physical examination, and the time spent with the patient. The number of diagnoses, management options, diagnostics and data, and the degree of medical risk are inclusive of medical decision making.

Coding of disorders and causes of death can be traced to the 17th century. The International Classification of Disease (ICD) was started in the 1900s in France. It originates from the international classification of causes of death, which was developed during a conference on the revision of the Bertillon. It listed 179 groups of causes of death and an abridged classification of 35 groups. In 1946 the responsibility for the ICD was transferred to the World Health Organization (WHO), which continually reviews and revises this classification system. Currently the ICD-10 is in use.

The Current Procedural Technology (CPT) code was developed by the American Medical Association (AMA) in 1966 and is revised and published yearly. It gives a descriptive term followed by a five-digit numeric number used for the reporting of medical services. These codes facilitate a standard communication between providers and payers.

The combination of ICD-10 and CPT codes yield the billable service. However, documentation must support the CPT code. Should the documentation not meet the required elements for billing, the health care provider can be charged with fraud. The Office of the Inspector General of the Department of Health and Human Services is responsible for prosecuting Medicare fraud. The electronic medical record is an efficient, time-reducing, and cost-containing method of documenting patient encounters. It allows for more readily available medical information and sharing, resulting in more thorough care of the patient. In addition, it allows accurate data to be generated by recording of exact times, resulting in improved departmental changes. In some programs, E&M coders can be activated to ensure that the proper billable documentation has been achieved. Institutions can share information with satellite sites as well as primary care providers and vice versa. This is essential as pertinent patient information would have been delayed or unobtainable in the past.

SUMMARY

Communication between health care providers and patients, obtaining consent, and accurate documentation provide the foundation for competent and thorough care. Providers should always take the time to listen and communicate with their patients. Discussion and education with patients provides a basis for realistic expectations and outcomes. Thorough and accurate documentation leads to decreased liability and fraud, resulting in accurate reimbursement: If it was not documented, it was not done.

Keeping patients informed throughout their care and thorough documentation make sense legally but more so ethically.

RESOURCES

Bitterman, R. A. (2010). Medicolegal issues and risk management. In J. A. Marx, R. S. Hockenberger, R. M. Walls, J. G. Adams, W. G. Barsan, M. H. Biros, et al. (Eds.), *Rosen's emergency medicine* (7th ed.). Retrieved from http://www.mdconsult.com/book/player/

book.do?method=display&type=bookPage&decorator=header&eid=4-u1.0-B978–0-323–05472-0..00202–4–s0200&displayedEid=4-u1.0-B978–0-323–05472-0..00202-4–s0205&uniq=187068169&isbn=978-0-323-05472-0&sid=962492495

CMS tightens documentation and signature requirements. Retrieved from http://www.health-carefinancenews.com/blog/cms-tightens-documentation-and-signature-requirements

International statistical classification of diseases and related health problems. *Encyclopedia of public health.* Retrieved from http://www.answers.com/topic/icd

Jawaid, S. A., & Jawaid, M. (2006). Patient's rights and the practice of obtaining informed consent: The need for some corrective measures. *Pakistan Journal of Medical Science, 22*(1), 7–9.

Loughlin, K. R. (2008). Medical malpractice: The good, the bad, and the ugly. *Urology Clinics of America, 36,* 101–110.

Medical documentation requirements. Retrieved from http://www.usbr.gov/mp/mp500/leave_share/medical_documentation_requirements.pdf

Medical liability reform. Retrieved from http://www.ama-assn.org/ama/pub/advocacy/current-topics-advocacy/practice-management/medical-liability-reform.shtml

Medical templates: Demystifying medical documentation. Retrieved from http://www.scribd.com/doc/7540597/Demystifying-Medical-Documentation

Medicare physician guide: A resource for residents, practicing physicians, and other health care professionals. (2009). *Department of Health and Senior Services.* Retrieved from http://gmc.sitcs.medinfo.ufl.edu/files/2010/03/Physician-Guide-to-Medicare-Services.pdf

Patient physician relationship topics: Informed consent. *American Medical Association.* Retrieved from http://www.ama-assn.org/ama/pub/physician-resources/legal-topics/patient-physician-relationship-topics/informed-consent.shtml on 12/1/9

Snyder, K. E., West, R. W., Lai, W. S., & Gay, S. B. Elements of informed consent. *University of Virginia health Sciences Center Department of Radiology.* Retrieved from http://www.med-ed.virginia.edu/courses/rad/consent/

Stern, T. A., Rosenbaum, J. F., Fava, M., Biederman, J., & Rauch, S. L. (2008). Informed consent, competency, treatment refusal, and civil commitment. *Massachusetts General Hospital Comprehensive Clinical Psychiatry.* Retrieved from http://www.mdconsult.com/das/book/body/187068169-6/962489283/1657/774.html#4-u1.0-B978-0-323–04743-2..50086 X–ccscc4_2389

Teichman, P. G. (2000). Documentation tips for reducing malpractice. *Family Practice Medicine.* Retrieved from http://www.aafp.org/fpm/20000300/29docu.html

3

Procedures for Basic Airway Management

KEITH A. LAFFERTY

BACKGROUND

While it is beyond the scope of this book to go into detail regarding formal and advanced airway management techniques, it behooves the provider who is performing minor surgical procedures using sedatives and potentially large doses of local anesthetics to have a fundamental understanding of basic airway maneuvers. Indeed, it is paramount for the provider to recognize potential airway compromise and act upon it early, before its sequelae of hypoxemia, acidosis, and obstruction may ensue.

Knowledge of the airway anatomy is mandatory. An appreciation of the importance of proper airway tone in maintaining airflow is crucial. Any decrease in consciousness, whether it be via trauma or iatrogenic medications, may allow the tongue to fall against the posterior pharyngeal wall, as well as induce a decrease in tone of the pharyngeal soft tissue. This causes a collapse of the hypopharynx and creates a partial and/or full airway occlusion.

PATIENT PRESENTATION

Signs of partial or complete airway obstruction include the following:

■ Decrease in mentation
■ Pooling of oral secretions
■ Stridor
■ Difficulty in phonation
■ Hypoxemia
■ Cyanosis

TREATMENT

Often, partial or complete airway obstruction can be overcome by simple techniques such as the chin lift, which overcomes lax musculature and tongue occlusion of the posterior pharynx, especially in the patient with a decreased level of consciousness.

A chin lift should be performed on every unconscious patient. This maneuver pulls the hyoid bone, anteriorly which in turn pulls the epiglottis and posterior tongue superiorly and anteriorly away from the posterior pharyngeal wall (Figure 3.1). Note

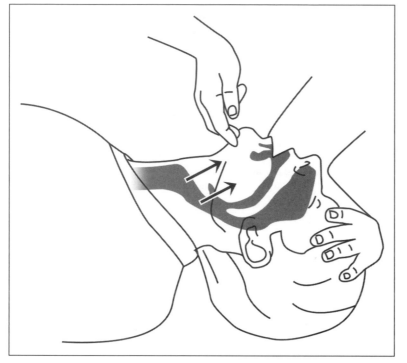

FIGURE 3.1
Sagittal view of chin lift
with airway anatomy.

that a child's airway demands greater attentiveness as children have a relatively larger tongue and smaller luminal airway diameter relative to adults.

SUPPLEMENTAL OXYGEN

Supplemental oxygenation (O_2) may be all that is required for patients in respiratory compromise, besides proper head positioning. The signs of hypoxemia include agitation, cyanosis, and change in heart rate. A pulse oximeter can be used to verify the above. Physiologically it is key to keep a patient's oxygen saturation near 100% because when it gets down to 90%, the corresponding PaO_2 is 60 mm Hg and is on the flat segment on the oxyhemoglobin dissociation curve. A further decrease will drop a patient's oxygenation exponentially.

Nasal Cannula

- Generally is better tolerated than a mask
- Can not deliver O_2 in excess of 3 L/min reliably
- Not a closed system, so the FiO_2 gain is only modest
- Further increases in flow cause nasal irritation and are not well tolerated by the patients

Simple O_2 Mask

- Delivers oxygen more readily than a nasal cannula
- Not as tolerable
- A minimum O_2 flow rate of 6 L/min must be maintained

■ Note, room air is allowed to enter the mask through exhalation ports and for this reason a Fio$_2$ of 35% to 60% is all that is delivered

Nonrebreather Mask

■ Contains one-way valves over the exhalation port, which allow egress of exhaled air while preventing the introduction of room air into the mask during inhalation
■ There is a one-way valve between the reservoir bag and the mask
■ Flow should be 10 to 12 L/min and a Fio$_2$ of 95% can be maintained

Bag Valve Mask

■ Must be utilized when all other methods fail
■ Experience lends a hand here as a tight seal is a must
■ Often used in conjunction with proper head positioning
■ May require an oral or nasopharyngeal airway
■ Tight seal is mandatory to prevent loss of air volume during ventilation
■ Problems encountered include inadequate tidal volume and gastric distention
■ An FIO$_2$ of 100% can be achieved with a proper seal

Suctioning

Occasionally, patient positioning and supplemental oxygen may be inadequate to achieve airway patency. Blood, vomitus, and secretions may require devices connected to tubing and wall suctioning to clear and maintain airway passage.

A soft catheter tip suction device may be used for gentle suction of the nasopharynx, especially for infants less than 6 months of age as they are obligate nasal breathers below this age. This can also be used to clear tracheostomy cannulas. They are not designed for suctioning thick secretions and/or particulate matter as the lumen can easily become occluded by such material.

The Yankauer or tonsil tip suction device is used to clear upper airway hemorrhage and secretions. A dental tip suction device may also be used and may offer a greater ability to remove particulate matter because its tip is not rounded like the Yankauer, although it may cause more pharyngeal trauma. Oral and pharyngeal suctioning should be performed in intervals no longer than 15 seconds to prevent further hypoxemia.

Complications of suctioning include the following:

■ Induction of vomiting
■ Possibility of creating a complete airway obstruction from a partial obstruction if material cannot be suctioned and becomes lodged
■ Bleeding
■ Pharyngeal wall injury
■ Brady dysrhythmias

Artificial Airways

Artificial airways must be used when basic head positions do not alleviate tongue/pharyngeal obstruction. These devices will bypass obstructive tissue, allowing for smooth nonturbulent airflow.

OROPHARYNGEAL AIRWAY

The oropharyngeal airway is limited in use to the unconscious patient as it causes pharyngeal irritation that can induce vomiting in the awake patient. It is composed of a piece of hard plastic with a central air channel and a flanged end that rests on the lips (Figure 3.2).

NASOPHARYNGEAL AIRWAY

The nasopharyngeal airway is among the simplest of artificial airways and its use is highly effective in preventing the tongue from falling back against the posterior pharyngeal wall and obstructing the airway. This device is less noxious than the oral pharyngeal airway in stimulating the gag reflex. It is made of a soft rubber material. Its size can be estimated by placing the flange end from the naris to the lobule of the ear. At this length it will rest just above the epiglottis (Figure 3.3).

PROCEDURE

Chin Lift

- Place the tips of the fingers beneath the patient's chin
- Lift the mandible forward

Bag Valve Mask

- Rescuers' hands must be large enough to apply pressure anteriorly by while simultaneously lifting the jaw forward
- The thumb and index finger provide anterior pressure while the fourth and fifth fingers lift the jaw placing pressure on the mandible not the soft tissue

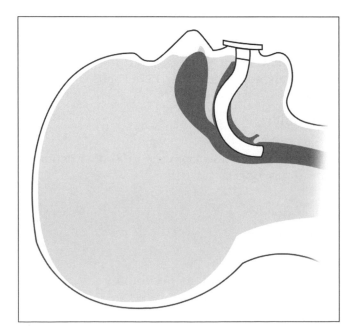

FIGURE 3.2 Proper insertion of an oropharyngeal airway.

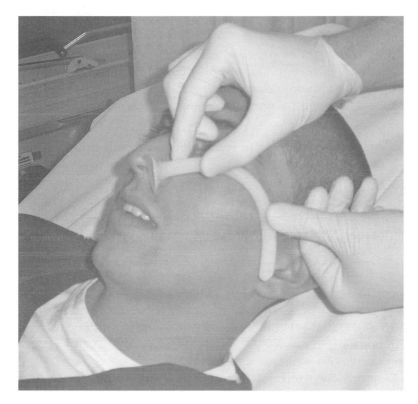

FIGURE 3.3
Nasopharyngeal
airway measurement.

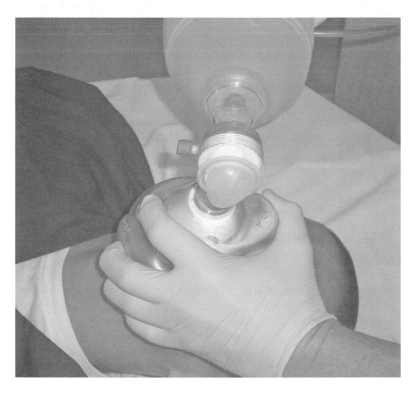

FIGURE 3.4 Bag valve
mask ventilation
technique.

- Complete compression of the bag must occur in order to give enough tidal volume for adequate ventilation (Figure 3.4)
- An assistant should apply firm posterior pressure on the cricoid ring in order to alleviate gastric inflation, although recent literature disputes this clinical dogma
- Dentures should be left in place to help ensure a better seal with the mask
- Attach tubing to supplemental oxygen with a flow rate of 15 L/min in order to prevent hypoxemia

Bag valve mask complications lead to inadequate ventilation and result from:

- A poor mask seal
- Failure to achieve proper airway patency
- Insufficient tidal volume
- Gastric distention can result from poor airway patency as air is insufflated in the esophagus and stomach with its inherent risk of regurgitation and aspiration

Oropharyngeal Airway

- Contraindicated in the awake patient
- Estimate proper size by placing it adjacent to the patient's face with the flange at the level of the anterior teeth and the distal component at the angle of the mandible
- Patient should be in supine position
- Tongue is depressed inferiorly with a tongue depressor
- Place the concave side inferiorly until the distal part rests in the posterior hypopharynx
- An alternative method would be to insert the device into the oral cavity in an inverted manner then rotate it 180° and advance until its distal end is pointed caudal in the hypopharynx
- This device essentially molds to the posterior tongue
- It separates the tongue from the posterior pharyngeal wall and pushes the epiglottis forward

COMPLICATIONS
- Vomiting
- If device is too small, it can push the epiglottis inferiorly, occluding the glottic opening
- If the device is too big, it can impinge and displace the tongue posteriorly and occlude the hypopharanyx (Figure 3.5)

Nasopharyngeal Airway

- Contraindicated in facial trauma
- Lubricate the device
- Place in the nostril of least resistance
- Insert posteriorly and toward the nasal septum
- May have to rotate upon placement
- If there is too much resistance, use other nostril

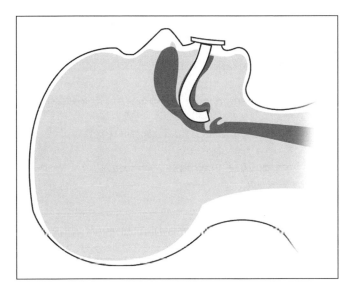

FIGURE 3.5 Incorrect size of oropharyngeal airway.

COMPLICATIONS
- Epistaxis
- Injury to nasal mucosa in adenoid tissue
- Sinusitis
- If device is too long, it can push epiglottis inferiority, occluding the glottic opening (Figure 3.6)
- In the face of a basiliar skull fracture, it may be inadvertently placed through the cribiform plate into the anterior cranial fossa

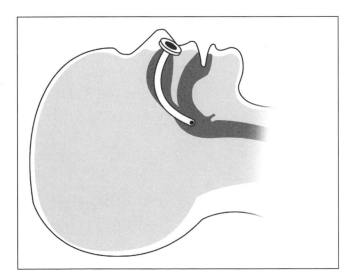

FIGURE 3.6 Incorrect size of an nasopharyngeal airway

AUTHOR'S PEARLS

- *Always use supplemental oxygen when administering sedatives or large amounts of local anesthetics*
- *The chin lift maneuver by itself commonly alleviates partial airway obstruction*
- *Routinely check resuscitation equipment and have it nearby for procedures involving sedatives or large doses of local anesthetics*
- *In almost all instances except teeth clenching, the nasopharyngeal airway is superior to the oropharyngeal airway*

RESOURCES

Bingham, R. M., & Proctor, L. T. (2008). Airway management. *Pediatric Clinics of North America, 55*, 873–886.

Bosson, N., & Gordon, P. E. (2009, March 6). Bag-valve-mask ventilation. Retrieved from http://emedicine.medscape.com/article/80184-overview

Clinton, J. E., & McGill, J. W. (2004). Basic airway management and decision-making. In J. Roberts & J. Hedges (Eds.), *Clinical procedures in emergency medicine* (pp. 53–68). Philadelphia: Saunders, Elsevier.

Lafferty, K. A., & Kulkarni, R. (2010, June 10). Tracheal intubation, rapid sequence intubation. Retrieved from http://emedicine.medscape.com/article/80222-overview & http://emedicine.medscape.com/article/80222-treatment

Santillanes, G. Pediatric airway management. *Emergency Medicine Clinics of North America, 24*(4), 961–975.

Scarfone, R. J. (2008). Oxygen delivery, suctioning, and airway adjuncts. In C. King & F. Henretig (Eds.), *Textbook of pediatric emergency procedures* (pp. 93–108). Philadelphia: Lippincott Williams & Wilkins.

4

Airway Foreign Body Removal

Keith A. Lafferty

BACKGROUND

Airway foreign bodies can be divided into upper (main bronchi and proximal) and lower (distal to main bronchi) impactions. More than 3,000 deaths occur annually secondary to foreign body aspirations; delayed presentation is common, outside of acute asphyxiation. Lower airway tract foreign bodies are a diagnostic challenge because of the following: 80% occur in children less than 3 years of age; the event is usually not witnessed and most foreign bodies are radiolucent such as peanuts, hot dogs, grapes, and so on. Because of this, one must maintain a high index of suspicion. In general, lower airway foreign bodies are not amenable to removal in the office or acute care setting. Note that, even though many signs are nonspecific at the initial presentation, 90% of children who have aspirated will give a history of choking, coughing, wheezing, or stridor. No doubt, recurrent croup, pneumonia, atelectasis, new onset asthma, pneumothorax, and pneumomediastinum should alert the clinician to arrange for a bronchoscopy, as this modality has decreased mortality from 50% to less than 1%. Even when the physical examination is unremarkable, if the history is possibly consistent with an acute aspiration (sudden symptoms or an object in the mouth that is suddenly missing) one must pursue this diagnosis.

Because more than two-thirds of aspirated foreign bodies are radiolucent, x-rays may show indirect evidence of their presence such as air trapping, mediastinal shift with expiration, atelectasis, pneumothorax, and pneumomediastinum. If the object is radiopaque, it may be seen oriented in the sagittal plane on the posteroanterior (PA) x-ray as the cartilaginous tracheal rings are not fused posteriorly.

The sudden and acute asphyxiation induced by a lodged upper airway foreign body (oralpharynx, hypopharynx, supraglottic, subglottic, or trachea) is a medical emergency. Any patient presenting with an acute upper airway aspiration who is not coughing, speaking, or displaying respiratory distress needs to be treated immediately. The cough reflex is the body's primary means of expelling a foreign body. This occurs via deep inspiration followed by a forced expiration against a closed glottis, which suddenly opens after high pressure forces it to do so. All immediate emergent treatments (Heimlich, back blow, and chest thrust maneuvers) essentially mimic this protective reflex. Patients presenting in this way should be treated as a 9-1-1 emergency, and standard basic life support/advanced life support (BLS/ALS) algorithms should be followed.

Further discussion will pertain to patients who present with a fish/chicken bone or pill foreign body sensation in their throat (Figure 4.1). As a rule, these

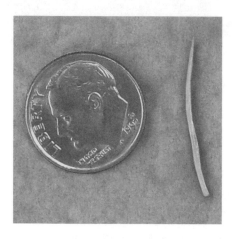

FIGURE 4.1 Fish bone. (Note the size in relation to a dime.)

patients are stable, give a clear history, and do not display any signs or symptoms of asphyxiation. They usually present immediately and can localize by pointing to the neck, where the foreign body sensation is felt. Indeed, most of these patients have a minor mucosal defect, which appears as a foreign body sensation. These usually heal within 24 hours.

Although most of the foreign bodies are in the hypopharynx, occasionally, with careful inspection with a tongue blade and light, some can be found in the oral pharynx (tonsils and base of the tongue). Clinically, the challenge is whether this is a foreign body or, more commonly, an abrasion. Adding to this diagnostic challenge is the following:

- Plain x-rays are less than 50% sensitive, as not all fish or chicken bones are radio-paque secondary to their high cartilagenous content (Figure 4.2)
- Less than 25% of patients who complain of a foreign body actually have it found endoscopically

The sensitivity of CT scans is more than 95% and they are widely available. Also, as a complementary modality, the nasopharyngeal laryngoscope (NPL) provides direct and complete visualization and is easy to use. Combining these two modalities essentially rules out the possibility of this diagnosis (Figure 4.3).

PATIENT PRESENTATION

- Patients usually present a few hours after the initial event
- They sit upright and often point with their finger to the area of the throat where the foreign body is felt
- They may experience odynophagia if the foreign body is placing pressure on the esophagus

TREATMENT

Treatment differs depending on the clinical setting and one's familiarization with fiber-optic equipment and/or the use of a laryngoscope. Patients are initially evaluated with a careful oropharyngeal inspection. If the foreign body can be identified

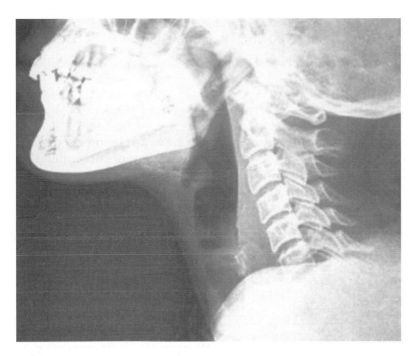

FIGURE 4.2 Lateral neck x-ray—note that the fishbone is not visualized.

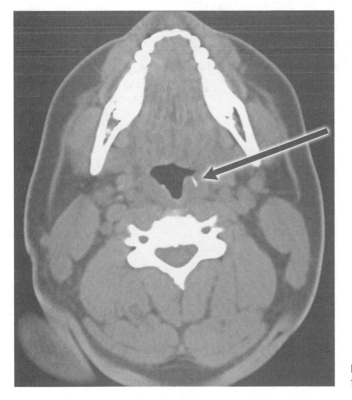

FIGURE 4.3 CT of the neck—the fishbone is radiopaque.

at this point and removed with forceps, the patient can be discharged. If further inspection is required, it usually includes the following modalities:

- Indirect laryngoscopy
- Direct laryngoscopy
- NPL
- CT scan

Fiberoptic visualization instruments, specifically the NPL, are being used with much more frequency in recent years. With a basic understanding of the upper airway anatomy, it is easily mastered with minimal practice. It is attached to a light source and inserted through the nares, through the nasopharynx, and into the hypopharynx. Its distal end moves superior and inferior with the control of a dial with the dominant hand. Its lateral movement is controlled with the nondominant hand holding the end just outside the patient's naris (Figures 4.4 and 4.5).

In recent years, because of much-increased sensitivity, CT scans have replaced plain x-rays and the NPL has replaced indirect laryngoscopy.

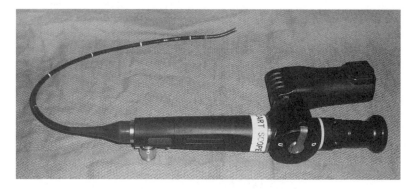

FIGURE 4.4
Nasopharyngeal laryngoscope (NPL).

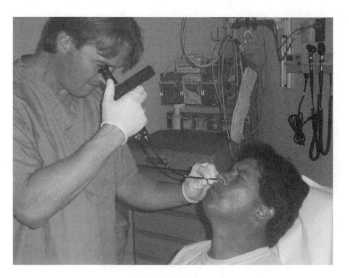

FIGURE 4.5 NPL technique.

CONTRAINDICATIONS

Unfamiliarity with the use of:

- NPL
- Laryngoscope

PROCEDURE PREPARATION

Indirect Laryngoscopy

- Laryngeal (dental) mirror
- Head lamp
- Gauze
- Benzocaine spray

Nasopharyngeal Laryngoscopy

- NPL
- Light source
- Benzocaine spray
- Water-based lubricant

Direct Laryngoscopy

- Laryngoscope and blade
- Benzocaine spray
- Viscous lidocaine
- Yankauer wall suction
- McGill forceps

PROCEDURE

Indirect Laryngoscopy

- Patient should sit in an upright position leaning slightly forward (sniffing position) with the head leaning back on a fixed surface to prevent head movement
- Spray the posterior pharynx with benzocaine
- Place the dental mirror in warm water to prevent condensation
- Wrap the tongue in gauze and grab it with the nondominant hand
- Place the mirror upside down in the posterior oropharynx and visualize the hypo-pharyngeal/supraglottic structures

Nasopharyngeal Laryngoscopy

- Patient should sit in an upright position leaning slightly forward (sniffing position) with the head leaning back on a fixed surface to prevent head movement
- Apply lubricant to the distal end of the NPL excluding the tip
- Spray the posterior pharynx with benzocaine
- Insert the NPL through the most patent naris (have the patient exhale through each naris separately while compressing the other) (Figure 4.5)

- Insert the NPL posteriorly past the turbinates and visualize the posterior pharynx, hypopharynx, and supraglottic and glottic structures (Figure 4.6)
- If fogging occurs, move the distal end to rub against the mucosa
- Have the patient say "e e e e," as this moves the vocal cords together and moves the glottis away from the larynx, providing a better view
- If a foreign body is seen, proceed to direct laryngoscopy

Direct Laryngoscopy

- After spraying the posterior pharynx with benzocaine, have the patient gargle for 1 minute three times with viscous lidocaine
- Patient should be lying on a stretcher in the supine position
- Provider should be standing at the head of the bed
- Check the light on the laryngoscope blade
- Using the left hand, place the laryngoscope blade along the floor of the mouth and gently lift up at a 45° angle
- Identify the foreign body and grasp with forceps

COMPLICATIONS

Retained Foreign Body

- Infection (retropharyngeal abscess)
- Asphyxiation

Indirect Laryngoscopy (Dental Mirror)

- Cough
- Vomiting

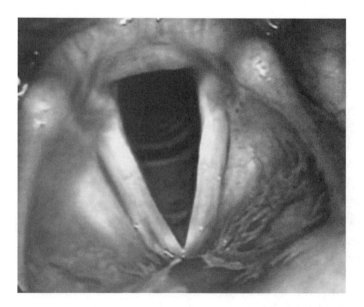

FIGURE 4.6 NPL visualization.

Nasopharyngeal Laryngoscopy

- Bleeding
- Abrasions
- Cough
- Vomiting

Direct Laryngoscopy

- Vomiting
- Bleeding
- Teeth trauma

AUTHOR'S PEARLS

- *Because of the low sensitivity of plain x-rays, x-rays can be eliminated in practices where an NPL and CT scan exist*
- *CT scans have a sensitivity of more than 95% in identifying fish/chicken bones*
- *If symptoms persist more than 24 hours, fiberoptic identification and extraction is indicated, as these usually will not dislodge and secondary bacterial infection will ensue*

RESOURCES

Cordle, R. (2004). Upper respiratory emergencies. In J. Tintinalli & G. Kelen (Eds.). *Emergency medicine: A comprehensive study guide* (pp.848–858). New York: McGraw-Hill.

Digoy, G. P. (2008). Diagnosis and management of upper aerodigestive tract foreign bodies. *Otolaryngology Clinics of North America, 41*(3), 485–496.

Munter, D. W., & Heffner, A. C. (2004). Esophageal foreign bodies. In J. Roberts & J. Hedges (Eds.), *Clinical procedures in emergency medicine* (pp. 775–793). Philadelphia: Saunders, Elsevier.

Riviello, R. J. (2004). Otolaryngologic procedures. In J. Roberts & J. Hedges (Eds.), *Clinical procedures in emergency medicine* (pp. 1280–1316). Philadelphia: Saunders, Elsevier.

Takada, M. (2000). 3D-CT diagnosis for ingested foreign bodies. *American Journal of Emergency Medicine, 18*(2), 192–193.

Thomas, S. H., & Brown, D. F. (2006). Foreign bodies. In J. Marx, R. Hockberger, & R. Walls (Eds.), *Rosen's emergency medicine concepts and clinical practice* (pp. 859–881). Philadelphia: Mosby, Elsevier.

5

Anesthetic Agents and Procedures for Local and Field Infiltration

KEITH A. LAFFERTY

BACKGROUND

The success rate of any procedure depends largely upon the modulation of pain. Ever since the first anesthetic agent was introduced in the late 1800s (cocaine), emergent procedures have progressed exponentially.

Pain fibers are peripheral nerves that begin at a receptor in the dermis and travel the length of the neuron ending at the spinal cord. Unlike thick, type A motor/pressure/proprioception nerve fibers, these thin type C pain fibers have no myelin sheath coverage and therefore are more susceptible to blockade by local anesthetics (LAs).

Although not fully understood, the mechanism of action of LAs has to do with the blockade of axonal nerve conduction. Normal neurons conduct an impulse by sodium influx via a specific sodium gate causing depolarization of the neuronal cell membrane, in a distal to proximal direction, to its articulation in the spinal cord. LAs, by either directly blocking sodium entry into the gate or by inducing swelling of the gate itself, do not allow depolarization and, therefore, no signal gets to the spinal cord and hence the brain (Figure 5.1).

Anesthetics are classified into two groups based on an intermediate chain that is either an esther or an amide. This intermediate chain is linked to an aromatic and a hydrophilic segment. The efficacy of each compound is directly related to the slight biochemical changes of these segments and dictates the time of onset, potency, and duration of actions of all the different agents. Metabolism occurs in esters via hydrolysis by plasma cholinesterases, while amides are degraded in the liver by microsomal enzymes.

Potency is directly proportional to liposolubility as the cell membranes that must penetrate and interact with the sodium channels are mostly composed of phospholipids. Time of onset has to do with how long it takes for an agent to reach the sodium channel. This is a property of its pKa, which is defined as the pH at which 50% of a structure is in both an ionized and an unionized form. So, the lower the pKa for a given LA and the higher the pH of the tissue it enters, the more availability of unionized molecules for cell membrane penetration. Finally, the duration of action relates to the level of protein binding that occurs at the receptor (see Table 5.1).

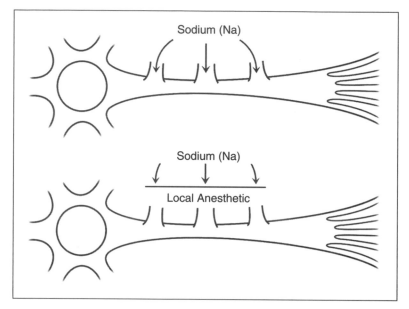

FIGURE 5.1 Neuron action potential— normal and blockade with LA.

TABLE 5.1 Anesthetic Agents—Onset, Duration, and Maximum Dose

Drug	Onset (minutes)	Duration (minutes)	Maximum Dose (mg/kg)
Procaine	5–10	30–60	7
Lidocaine			
Without epinephrine	2–5	30–120	4
With epinephrine	2–5	60–180	7
Bupivicaine			
Without epinephrine	5–10	180–360	2
With epinephrine	5–10	240–600	3
Mepivacaine	2–5	90–180	6
Diphenhydramine	2–5	20–30	1.5

Certain characteristics have been shown to decrease injection pain:

- Slow injection (causes less distention of tissue)
- Keeping the solution warm (40°C)
- Adding a bicarbonate buffer in a 1:10 ratio with the amides (the esters will precipitate)

Adding epinephrine to the LA allows a larger dose to be used, as epinephrine induces local vasoconstriction and decreases systemic absorption. Note that there is no evidence that this has any negative effect on end arterial areas.

LAs interact with sodium gates of neuronal tissue and also of all excitable tissues (any cell membrane possessing the ability to depolarize). The central nervous

TABLE 5.2 Signs and Symptoms of Toxicity

Central Nervous System	Cardiovascular System	Neuromuscular Junction
Slurring	Premature ventricular contractions	Paresthesias
Tinnitus	Bradydysarhythmias	Tremor
Confusion	Heart blocks	Twitching
Seizures	Hypotension	Myoclonic jerks

system (CNS), cardiovascular (CV) system, and neuromuscular junction (NMJ) are susceptible to its action and toxicity, especially when high plasma levels are reached. Adding to the CNS susceptibility is the fact that these agents are so lipophilic and cross the blood-brain barrier easily. Other mechanisms contributing to CV toxicity is the fact that LAs are negative inotropes and that they decrease the peripheral vascular resistance. Note that many antidysrhythmics interacting with sodium gates should not be used in cases of CV toxicity. Bretylium is the antidysrhythmic drug shown to be most effective. Lesion-specific anticonvultants like phenytoin are ineffective for seizures. In general, sympathomimetics should be utilized (e.g., benzodiazapines, diprovan). Signs and symptoms of toxicity do occur in a stepwise manner for the given organ system involved (see Table 5.2).

Although much talked about, true allergic reactions are extremely rare. If they do occur, it is usually from an ester compound. A degradation product of the esters is para-amino benzoic acid (PABA), which is responsible for the majority of the allergic reactions. Amides are stored in a solution containing methylparaben, which is similar in composition and antigenicity to PABA. If one truly has an ester allergy, use of the code cart lidocaine, which is devoid of methylparaben, can be an option. Also, if unsure of the class to which a patient is allergic, diphenhydramine can be used for injection after diluting to a 1% solution (10 mg/mL).

TREATMENT

Local anesthesia for wound management is delivered via three different techniques:

- Topical anesthesia
- Infiltrative anesthesia
- Field block anesthesia

Topical Anesthesia

This can be applied upon arrival while the patient is awaiting evaluation and treatment by the provider. Topical anesthesia (TA) has been shown to decrease the need for infiltrative anesthesia. Smaller lacerations or multiple localized abrasions (road rash) may be amenable to this therapy. Although this displays a low potency and a delayed onset, its attributes include easy application, potential decrease in need for child restraints, and no distortion of wound edges.

- TAC (tetracaine, adrenaline, cocaine)—replaced by less toxic preparations
- LET (lidocaine, epinephrine, tetracaine)—as effective as TAC

■ Ethyl chloride and fluori-methane sprays—vapor coolants; upon topical application, the skin is cooled to −20°C, temporarily freezing the skin (less than 1 minute)
■ Benzocaine—highly insoluble in water; used on the mucous membranes

Infiltrative Anesthesia

This is the mainstay of wound anesthesia. It has rapid onset with low systemic toxicity. Injection at the wound margin induces less pain than through the epidermis without an increase in the infection rate. Pinching of the skin at the time of injection has been shown to decrease the pain. A 25- or 27-gauge needle should be used as smaller lumens induce too much injection resistance. Placement of the needle just below the dermis at the level of the superficial fascia is less painful than placement in the dermis, and offers less tissue resistance as the fascia is composed of loose connective and adipose tissue.

Field Block Anesthesia

A subcutaneous layer of LA is placed at an area away from the wound, surrounding the wound with a linear parallel wall of the agent. This can be used in areas such as the ear, where infiltrative anesthesia would be an anatomical challenge. This may also be used in largely contaminated wounds. Although multiple needle sticks through the epidermis are required, pain can be decreased by administration of subsequent LA through previously anesthetized skin.

The maximal dose of the LA can be calculated as follows: For a 70-kg patient being given lidocaine with epinephrine (max dose 7 mg/kg):

■ A 100% solution is 1 g/mL or 1,000 mg/mL so a 1% solution is 10 mg/mL
■ Maximal dose is 490 mg or 49 mL

CONTRAINDICATIONS

■ Allergy

PROCEDURE PREPARATION

■ Supine or comfortable position of the patient
■ LA should be administered before formal wound irrigation/cleansing

Topical Anesthesia

■ Gloves
■ Sterile cotton ball or gauze
■ LET (lidocaine 4%, epinephrine 0.1%, tetracaine 0.5%)

Infiltrative Anesthesia and Field Block Anesthesia

■ Gloves
■ Skin cleanser
■ LA
■ Syringe
■ 25- or 27-gauge needle

PROCEDURE

Topical Anesthesia

- Remove gross decontaminants
- Soak cotton ball or gauze and sprinkle drops over the wound
- Apply applicant with an occlusive dressing
- Allow at least 30 minutes for effect

Infiltrative Anesthesia

- Direct the needle into the wound margin just below the dermis at the level of the superficial fascia (Figure 5.2)
- Insert the needle two-thirds of its length and advance in a direction that is parallel to the wound edge
- Inject the LA upon slow withdrawal of the needle
- Repeat this step in an area where the LA was previously deposited

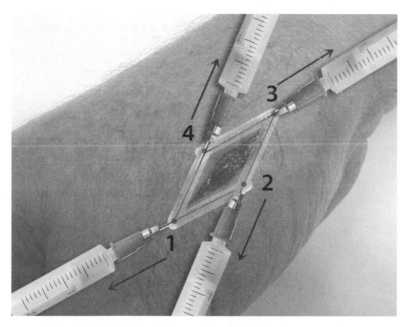

FIGURE 5.2
Infiltrative anesthesia technique.

Field Block Anesthesia

- Insert the needle 1 cm away from the wound or structure through the epidermis to the level of the subcutaneous tissue (superficial fascia)
- Insert the needle two-thirds of its length and advance in a direction that is parallel to the wound edge
- Inject the LA upon slow withdrawal of the needle
- Continue repetition of the previous step until a wall of LA is deposited around the wound or a diamond shape surrounds the structure (e.g., when applying to the ear)
- Repeated injections should be placed in an area where the LA was previously deposited (Figure 5.3)

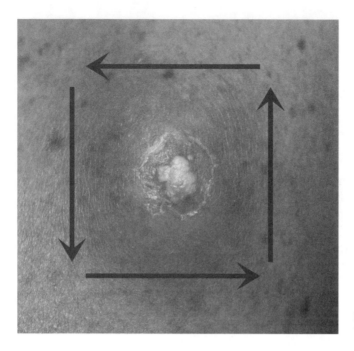

FIGURE 5.3 Field block anesthesia technique.

COMPLICATIONS

- Infection
- Bleeding
- CV toxicity
- CNS toxicity
- Vasovagal syncope

Author's Pearls

- *Bupivicaine last longer than lidocaine*
- *True allergic reaction consists of urticaria, pruritis, wheezing, and so on and not vasovagal symptoms*
- *Use LA liberally, even in wounds without a closure, as there is no reason to inflict unnecessary pain to patients*
- *Injection through the wound edges is less painful than through the epidermis*
- *Topical agents are well tolerated and effective in children*
- *Though most cases of systemic toxicity are caused by inadvertent intravenous injection, calculate the maximal dose for large wounds*
- *A quick method for converting any LA concentration is to add a zero after the numerical percent—a 1% solution is 10 mg/mL*

RESOURCES

Crystal, C. S. (2007). Anesthetic and procedural sedation techniques for wound management. *Emergency Med Clinics of North America, 25*(1), 41–71.

Harmatz, A. (2009). Local anesthetics: Uses and toxicities. *Surgery Clinics of North America, 89*(3), 587–598.

Higginbothan, E., & Vissers, R. J. (2004). Local and regional anesthesia. In J. Tintinalli & G. Kelen (Eds.), *Emergency medicine: A comprehensive study guide* (pp. 264–274). New York: McGraw-Hill.

Jackson, T. (2006). Pharmacology of local anesthetics. *Ophthalmologic Clinics of North America, 19*(2), 155–161.

Kapitanyan, R., & Su, M. (2009). Toxicity, local anesthetics. Retrieved from http://emedicine.medscape.com/article/819628-overview

McCreight, A., & Stephan, M. (2008). Local and regional anesthesia. In C. King & F. Henretig (Eds.), *Textbook of pediatric emergency procedures* (pp. 439–469). Philadelphia: Lippincott Williams & Wilkins.

Paris, P. M., & Yealy, D. M. (2006). Pain management. In J. Marx, R. Hockberger, & R. Walls (Eds.), *Rosen's emergency medicine concepts and clinical practice* (pp. 2913–2937). Philadelphia: Mosby, Elsevier.

6

Procedures for Performing Regional Anesthesia

KEITH A. LAFFERTY

BACKGROUND

Blocking a peripheral nerve is intuitively more advantageous because the nerve is inhibited before its distal tributaries. A digital nerve block is the most common use of this technique and is discussed in Chapter 7.

Advantages of regional anesthesia over infiltrative anesthesia include the following:

- Broad area covered
- Less local anesthetic (LA) administered

Also, some areas of the body such as the ear, palm, sole, and so on, are not amenable to infiltrative anesthesia. In the case of the plantar foot, the large amount of sensory fibers combine and with the difficulty of injecting through the dense, septated connective tissue makes regional anesthesia a prudent choice.

These nerve blocks are not as easily mastered as the infiltrative anesthesia technique. However, with repetition, a continued review of the peripheral neuroanatomy, and proper training and supervision, one can gain comfort and success with such procedures.

Nerve blocks more proximal to the wrist and ankle, with the exception of an intercostal and penile block, will not be discussed as they are more often used in the operating room and may require a nerve stimulator or an ultrasound machine to precisely localize them. Also, bupivicaine is recommended over lidocaine because of its longer duration of action in general.

PATIENT PRESENTATION

Use with any patient presenting with an injury distal to the nerve being anesthetized, such as:

- Laceration
- Abscess
- Fracture
- Dislocation
- Burns

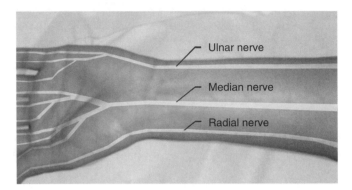

FIGURE 6.1 Ulnar, radial, and median nerves—volar wrist.

TREATMENT

Ulnar Nerve Block

The ulnar nerve supplies sensation to the medial third of the dorsal hand, small finger, and the ulnar half of the ring finger. The ulnar nerve runs along the volar aspect of the wrist, bordered medially by the ulnar artery and laterally by the flexor carpi ulnaris. Note that it lies just deep to this tendon flexor, making a volar approach difficult (Figures 6.1–6.3). Identification of the proximal carpi ulnaris at the proximal palmar crease is simplified by having the patient flex the wrist against resistance.

Radial Nerve Block

Proximal to the wrist, the radial nerve has already divided into tributaries that enter the radial aspect of the wrist. Sensation is provided in the lateral two-thirds of the dorsal hand, the proximal dorsal thumb, index, long, and the radial half of the fourth finger. Note that the nail beds of the fingers are supplied by the median nerve, which makes up half of the dorsal digital nerve (Figures 6.1–6.3).

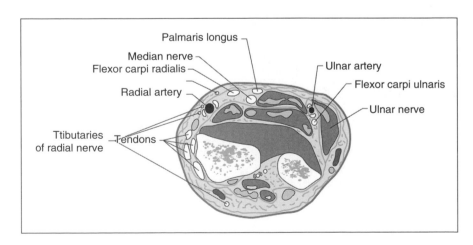

FIGURE 6.2 Cross-section—wrist.

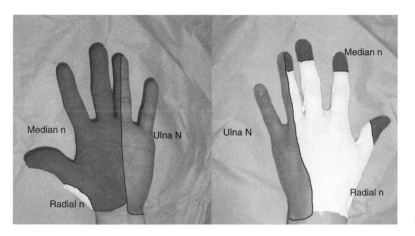

FIGURE 6.3
Dermatones of the hand.

Median Nerve Block

The median nerve provides sensation to the lateral two-thirds of the palm. It also supplies the distal dorsal thumb, the index and middle fingers, and the lateral half of the distal ring finger. The median nerve at the wrist is bordered medially by the palmaris longis tendon and laterally by the flexor carpi radialis at a depth just below the former tendon. Note that 20% of the population may be without the palmaris longis tendon. The palmaris longis is identified by having the patient oppose their thumb and small finger in wrist flexion with resistance. Note that the flexor carpi radialis is just lateral to this (Figures 6.1–6.3).

Posterior Tibial Nerve and Sural Blocks

The posterior tibial nerve and the sural nerve are tributaries of the tibial nerve. The posterior tibial nerve supplies the majority of the plantar surface sensation, along with the sural nerve medially and the saphenous nerve laterally. The posterior tibial nerve runs along the medial aspect of the ankle just deep and posterior to the posterior tibial artery between the medial malleolus and the Achilles tendon. It is identified by palpating the posterior tibial artery, which is located just posteriorly to the medial malleolus. The sural nerve runs subcutaneously between the lateral malleolus and the Achilles tendon. Often, these two nerves are blocked simultaneously to anesthetize the plantar surface entirely—a posterior ankle block (Figures 6.4–6.6).

Intercostal Nerve Block

This is one of the most underused nerve blocks. The fear of causing an iatrogenic pneumothorax is unwarranted as the incidence is less than 0.1%. Rib fractures, contusions, and post–chest tube thoracostomy are ideal candidates. Although the duration of action of long-acting LAs is 8 to 12 hours, patients get continued relief for up to 3 days with this procedure. It should be noted that the intercostal nerve block has the potential for rapid vascular absorption though doses used are well below toxic levels. Care must be taken to correctly calculate the maximum dose of LA, though typically this is not

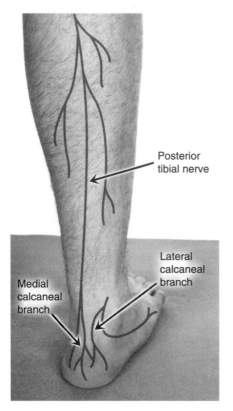

Posterior
tibial nerve

Lateral
calcaneal
branch

Medial
calcaneal
branch

FIGURE 6.4 Posterior tibial nerves.

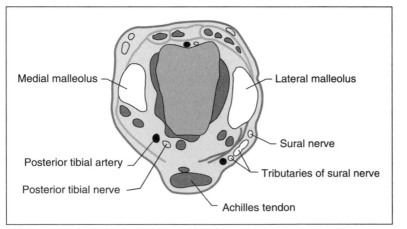

Medial malleolus

Lateral malleolus

Sural nerve

Posterior tibial artery

Tributaries of sural nerve

Posterior tibial nerve

Achilles tendon

FIGURE 6.5 Cross-section—ankle.

reached. This minimizes the splinting associated with rib injuries and its sequelae of atelectasis and pneumonia.

The intercostal groove accommodates, in a superior to inferior manner, the intercostal vein, artery, and nerve. Posteriorly, it is separated from the pleural space

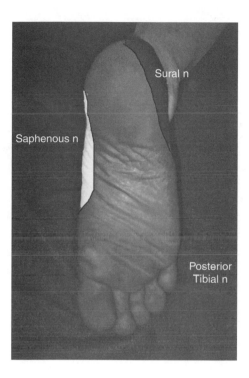

FIGURE 6.6 Dermatone of plantar foot.

by only a thin intercostal fascia. Laterally, it is sandwiched between the internal and external intercostal muscles. The entry point of the needle should be at the inferior border of the rib on the lateral chest wall. A postprocedure chest x-ray is not needed (Figure 6.7).

Penile Block

The two dorsal nerves of the penis supply each half of the dorsal glands and shaft. They lie just off the midline at the 10 and 2 o'clock positions at the base of the shaft. They are just deep to the fibrous buck's fascia. The anterior surface is supplied by cutaneous sacral plexus nerves. Because of this, nerve blocks can anesthetize the dorsal penis, whereas a ring block must be used to anesthetize the anterior penis.

PROCEDURE PREPARATION

- Wrist blocks are best accomplished with the patient in the supine position with the forearm/wrist resting with the volar surface
- Posterior ankle blocks are best positioned with the patient prone and the ankle hanging off the end of the stretcher with the foot in slight dorsiflexion

CONTRAINDICATIONS

- Allergy
- Compartment syndrome

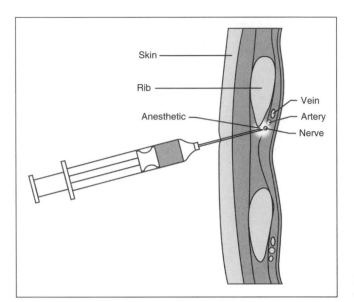

FIGURE 6.7 Intercostal groove contents—inferior rib border.

PROCEDURE

Ulnar Nerve Block

- Insert a 25-gauge needle horizontally into the medial wrist just under the flexor carpi ulnaris at the level of the proximal palmar crease (Figure 6.8)
- Inject 5 mL of the LA
- Inject a subcutaneous partial ring block from the lateral border of the flexor carpi ulnaris and continue medially to the dorsal half of the wrist in order to anesthetize cutaneous fibers

Radial Nerve Block

- Insert a 25-gauge needle horizontally into the lateral wrist until it is just lateral to the radial artery at the level of the palmar crease (Figure 6.8)
- Inject 5 mL of the LA
- Inject a subcutaneous partial ring block from this lateral entry point and continue laterally to the dorsal half of the wrist in order to anesthetize cutaneous fibers

Median Nerve Block

- Insert a 27-gauge needle perpendicular to the skin between the palmaris longis and the flexor carpi radialis at the level of the proximal palmar crease (Figure 6.8)
- Inject 5 mL of the LA

Posterior Tibial Nerve Block

- Insert a 25-gauge needle at a 45-degree angle anteriorly just posterior to the posterior tibial artery at the level of the superior surface of the medial malleolus (Figure 6.9)
- Inject 5 mL of the LA
- If no paresthesia elicited, direct the needle in a more perpendicular direction

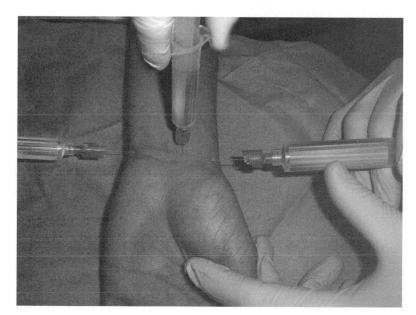

FIGURE 6.8 Needle entry point for wrist blocks.

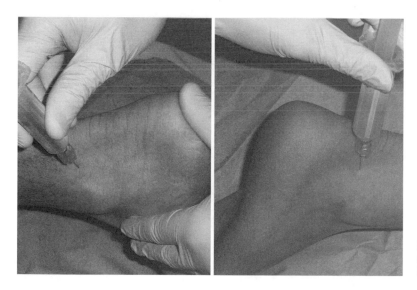

FIGURE 6.9 Needle entry point for ankle blocks.

Sural Nerve Block

- Insert a 25-gauge needle anteriorly between the Achilles tendon and the lateral malleolus about 1 cm superior to the lateral malleolus (Figure 6.9)
- Inject 5 mL of the LA
- Inject a subcutaneous partial field block between the Achilles and the lateral malleolus in order to anesthetize cutaneous fibers

Intercostal Nerve Block

- Patient should be sitting upright with legs hanging off the side of the stretcher
- Insert a 25-gauge needle perpendicular to the skin between the mid and posterior axillary line directly
- After striking the rib with the needle, retract the needle slightly (without withdrawing completely) and readvance in a slightly more inferior position in an attempt to "walk" the needle down the rib
- At a point just below the intercostal groove, advance the needle 3 mm beyond the inferior border (Figure 6.10)
- Inject 5 mL of the LA
- Repeat this procedure for one or two ribs above and below the site of injury in order to anesthetize cross innervation

Penile Block

- Insert a 25-gauge needle perpendicular to the abdominal wall, at the base of the penis at the 10 and 2 o'clock positions
- Inject 5 mL of the LA in both sides
- The depth of the needle should be 0.5 cm below the skin. One may feel a "pop" as buck's facia is penetrated
- Inject a subcutaneous partial ring block around the posterior base of the penis

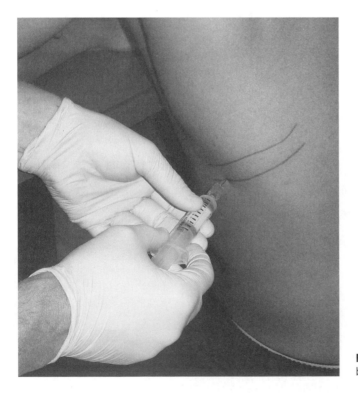

FIGURE 6.10 Intercostal nerve block.

COMPLICATIONS

- Infection
- Bleeding
- Peripheral nerve injury
- Compartment syndrome
- Cardiovascular toxicity
- Central nervous system toxicity
- Vasovagal syncope

AUTHOR'S PEARLS

- *Allow at least 15 minutes for effect, and more time if the injury is more distal to the block*
- *Epinephrine allows the LA to remain near the nerve longer and increases the duration of action*
- *Eliciting distal paresthesia with the needle before injection implies contact with the nerve*
- *Keep in mind that some structures have secondary cutaneous innervation (i.e., hand and penis) and note the importance of a circumferential ring block to complement the primary target nerve*
- *Dual nerves in some structures [that is, the wrist (radial and ulnar)], may be required for a particular area to receive full anesthesia*
- *Intercostal nerve blocks are safe and offer significant relief of pain*

RESOURCES

Crystal, C. S. (2007). Anesthetic and procedural sedation techniques for wound management. *Emergency Medicine Clinics of North America, 25*(1), 41–71.

Higginbothan, E., & Vissers R. J. (2004). Local and regional anesthesia. In J. Tintinalli & G. Kelen (Eds.), *Emergency medicine: A comprehensive study guide* (pp. 264–274). New York: McGraw-Hill.

McCreight, A., & Stephan, M. (2008). Local and regional anesthesia. In C. King & F. Henretig (Eds.), *Textbook of pediatric emergency procedures* (pp. 439–469). Philadelphia: Lippincott Williams & Wilkins.

Morgan, G. E., & Mikhail, M. S. (2002). Peripheral nerve blocks. In G. E. Morgan, M. S. Mikhail, & M. J. Murray (Eds.), *Clinical anesthesiology* (3rd ed., pp. 283–308). New York: Lange Medical Books.

Simon, B., & Hern, G. (2006). Wound management principals. In J. Marx, R. Hockberger, & R. Walls (Eds.), *Rosen's emergency medicine concepts and clinical practice* (pp. 845–846). Philadelphia: Mosby, Elsevier.

Procedure for Performing Digital Anesthesia

KEITH A. LAFFERTY

BACKGROUND

By far, a digital nerve block is the most commonly used regional nerve block in the outpatient setting. It provides fast, effective, and simple anesthesia. Because the structure of the distal finger has fibrous septations, local infiltrative anesthesia is not only impractical but also nearly impossible.

As in most procedures, the key to a successful outcome is a fundamental understanding of the anatomy. A common digital nerve runs along the side of the metacarpals and, at the level of the metacarpal heads, bifurcates into volar and dorsal tributaries.

The end result is that there are lateral, dorsal, and medial digital nerves as well as their radial counterparts. Specifically, they lay along side the phalanx at the 2, 10, 4, and 8 o'clock positions. Dorsal fibers are derived from the radial and ulnar nerves, whereas volar fibers stem from the median and ulnar nerves. Although both a dorsal and palmar approach can be used, the former is more desirable as it has less subcutaneous pain fibers. The innervation of the toes follows a similar pattern.

A metacarpal nerve block that is more proximal can be used as well before the bifurcation at the metacarpal head. Its advantage is that it provides more proximal anesthesia; however, it is more difficult and occasionally less effective.

The thumb and hallux (great toe) have accessory nerves running over the dorsal lateral surface, much more so than the other digits. Because of this, the provider should make a circumferential subcutaneous ring pattern with the local anesthetic.

PATIENT PRESENTATION

Digital pathology of the finger/toe, including the following:

- Lacerations
- Paronychia
- Nail bed injuries
- Fracture
- Dislocation
- Ring removal
- Tendon injuries

TREATMENT

Local anesthetic injection should occur at least 10 minutes before the procedure to allow complete anesthesia. Although it is commonly stated that epinephrine should not be used, there is no evidence supporting this. In fact, according to current evidence, the use of epinephrine with lidocaine in standard commercial concentrations for digital blocks is not harmful and is likely advantageous, as epinephrine with lidocaine decreases the use of tourniquets and repeated sticks.

CONTRAINDICATIONS

■ Compartment syndrome of the finger

PROCEDURE PREPARATION

■ Patient should be supine with the finger well exposed and comfortably resting on the table
■ Skin antiseptic solution
■ Bupivacaine or lidocaine
■ 25- or 27-gauge needle

PROCEDURE

■ Skin cleansing technique as described in Chapter 10
■ Sterile technique
■ The volar surface of the hand is placed on the table
■ The needle is inserted at a 90° angle in the dorsal hand at the level of the web space along the proximal phalynx tenting the volar skin
■ Upon slow withdrawal of the needle, 2 mL of local anesthetic is deposited
■ Just before needle withdrawal from the skin, a 1 cc deposit is injected in the dorsal surface of the finger
■ The needle is reinserted in the other side of the finger through the anesthetized dorsal surface as described previously (Figure 7.1)

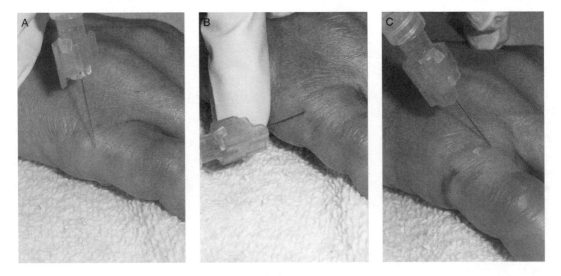

FIGURE 7.1 Digital nerve block insertion sites.

AUTHOR'S PEARLS

■ *Allow adequate time for onset of this peripheral nerve block—at least 10 minutes*
■ *Bupivacaine lasts longer than lidocaine*
■ *The finger tips are not amenable to the infiltrate of local anesthesia secondary to fibrous septae*

RESOURCES

Kelly, J. J., & Spektor, M. (2004). Nerve blocks of the thorax and extremities. In J. Roberts & J. Hedges (Eds.), *Clinical procedures in emergency medicine* (pp. 567–590). Philadelphia: Saunders.

McCreight, A., & Stephan, M. (2008). Local and regional anesthesia. In C. King & F. Henretig (Eds.), *Textbook of pediatric emergency procedures* (pp. 439–464). Philadelphia: Lippincott Williams & Wilkins.

Volfson, D. (January 27, 2010). Anesthesia, regional, digital block. Retrieved from http://emedicine.medscape.com/article/80887-overview

Waterbrook, A. L. (2007). Is epinephrine harmful when used with anesthetics for digital nerve blocks? *Annals of Emergency Medicine, 50*(4), 472–475.

8

Procedure for Performing Beir Anesthesia

KEITH A. LAFFERTY

BACKGROUND

This technique was first described in 1908 and has withstood the test of time, although it is much underused. This type of venous anesthesia involves IV infusion of a local anesthetic (LA) in the distal extremity via the proximal part constricted via a pneumatic tourniquet. The LA is forced to permeate the venous walls and capillaries and to remain in the portion of the extremity distal to the pneumatic cuff, which has a higher pressure than the systolic blood pressure. The technique allows rapid onset of limb anesthesia (paresis), provides a bloodless field, and is safe, and effective, and easy to perform. Although this involves a large dose of an LA intravenously, a recent review in the literature shows no mortality and very little morbidity.

Different mechanisms of action probably contribute to its overall effect. Besides the sodium channel blockade theory, ischemia and acidosis probably contribute to the anesthesia, as prior to the discovery of LAs, surgical procedures were carried out just with pneumatic compression of nerve tunnels.

PATIENT PRESENTATION

- Large extremity lacerations (repair)
- Extremity fractures (reduction)
- Extremity dislocations (reduction)
- Extremity burns (debridement)
- Extremity abscess incision and drainage
- Extremity tendon lacerations (repair)

TREATMENT

Because the position of the pneumatic cuff overlies the proximal extremity, this procedure is best used for injuries at or below the elbow and knee. The area is exsanguinated before the procedure begins in order to maintain a bloodless field. A key feature of this procedure is that all of the LA is contained in the extremity and does not enter the systemic circulation. Two pneumatic cuffs are used—a proximal and a distal. The proximal cuff is inflated first and only after onset of anesthesia distal to this cuff is reached, then the distal cuff is inflated and the proximal cuff is deflated. This is done to decrease the pain induced by the cuff pressure.

Lidocaine is chosen over bupivacaine because it is less cardiac toxic and may remain active after cuff deflation. The concentration of lidocaine to be used is 0.5%. Although the literature states that lidocaine can be used at a dose of 3 mg/kg, a mini dose of 1.5 mg/kg can be used with similar efficacy and less potential toxicity. If needed, repeat doses of 0.5 mg/kg can be given. Expected onset is 5 to 10 minutes in a progression of paresthesia, anesthesia to paresis in a distal to proximal manner.

CONTRAINDICATIONS

■ Raynaud's disease
■ Homozygous sickle cell disease
■ Significant cardiac disease
■ Unreliable tourniquet

PROCEDURE PREPARATION

■ Patient should be supine on the stretcher
■ An IV is placed in the ipsilateral extremity for the LA
■ Another IV is placed in the contralateral extremity for the administration of resuscitation medications if needed
■ Two pneumatic tourniquets
■ Elastic bandage
■ Cardiac monitor with pulse oximeter
■ Resuscitation cart in room
■ Lidocaine 0.5% without epinephrine
■ Large syringe for the lidocaine injection

PROCEDURE

■ Place the patient in a supine position on cardiac monitor and pulse oximeter
■ Place IV in both extremities
■ Exsanguinate the extremity via arm raising and Ace-wrap compression in a distal to proximal manner
■ Inflate the proximal pneumatic cuff to 100 mm Hg above the patient's systolic blood pressure
■ Remove Ace wrap
■ Inject lidocaine at a dose of 1.5 mg/kg over 1 minute (Figure 8.1)
■ At onset of effect, inflate the distal cuff and deflate the proximal cuff in order to decrease cuff-induced pain
■ Rebolus 0.5 mg/kg of lidocaine if needed
■ After completion of procedure, deflate the cuff for 10 seconds and then reinflate. Do this for three cycles.

COMPLICATIONS

These are rare and usually result from an improper and malfunctioning tourniquet and subsequent release of a large bolus of the LA into the systemic circulation. Treatment is with standard resuscitation techniques; however, it should be noted that

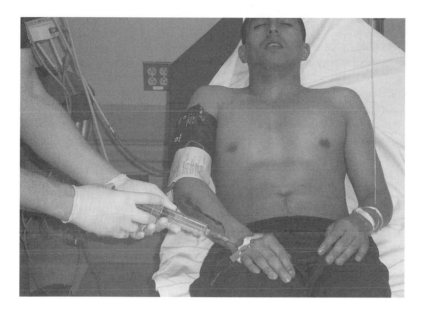

FIGURE 8.1 Bier block.

benzodiazepines treat most of these signs and symptoms. If this occurs, observe the following signs/symptoms:

- Nausea
- Vomiting
- Dizziness
- Tinnitus
- Brady dysarhythmias
- Decreased mentation
- Scizurcs

Author's Pearls

- *It is of paramount importance to repeatedly check and maintain proper cuff inflation throughout the procedure*
- *Use the mini dose of lidocaine (1.5 mg/kg instead of the standard 3 mg/ kg dose) as it has similar efficacy but less toxicity if systemic release occurs*
- *If used on the lower extremity, the cuff should not be higher than the mid-calf to prevent peroneal nerve injury*
- *Confirm the absence of a radial pulse before injection of the LA*
- *Skin blanching after the injection of the LA is normal and probably a result of blood extravasation from capillaries as it is being displaced by the LA*
- *If 0.5% lidocaine cannot be found, it can be made from a 1% solution by creating a 50/50 solution with normal saline*

RESOURCES

Bolte, R. G., & Stevens, P. M. (1994). Mini-dose bier block intravenous regional anesthesia in the emergency department treatment of pediatric upper-exremity injuries. *Journal of Pediatric Orthopaedics, 14*(4), 534–537.

Guay, J. (2009). Adverse events associated with intravenous regional anesthesia (Bier block): A systematic review of complications. *Journal of Clinical Anesthesia, 21*(8), 585–594.

McCreight, A., & Stephan, M. (2008). Local and regional anesthesia. In C. King & F. Henretig (Eds.), *Textbook of pediatric emergency procedures* (pp. 439–468). Philadelphia: Lippincott Williams & Wilkins.

Mohr, B. (2006). Safety and effectiveness of intravenous regional anesthesia (Bier block) for outpatient management of forearm trauma. *Canadian Journal of Emergency Medicine, 8*(4), 247–250.

Procedure for Performing Auricular Anesthesia

Theresa M. Campo

BACKGROUND

Auricular blocks can be used to treat extensive lacerations and auricular hematomas, and other painful procedures to the external ear.

The ear, also known as the auricle, is divided into three areas: external, middle, and internal structures. Discussion will be limited to the external auricle in this book. The external ear is innervated by four branches of nerves: (1) the greater auricular nerve (branches off from the cervical plexus), (2) lesser occipital nerve, (3) auricular branch of the vagus nerve, and (4) auriculotemporal nerve (Table 9.1 and Figure 9.1).

CONTRAINDICATIONS AND RELATIVE CONTRAINDICATIONS

- Cellulitis
- Severe allergy to anesthetic agent

TABLE 9.1 Auricular Nerve Branch and Innervation

Nerve Branch	Innervation
Greater auricular nerve (branch of cervical plexus)	Auricle Posteromedial Posterolateral Inferior
Lesser occipital nerve (branch of cervical plexus)	Few branches may contribute to: Auricle Posteromedial Posterolateral Inferior
Auricular branch of vagus nerve (cranial nerve [CN] X)	Concha Most of the auditory meatus tympanic membrane
Auriculotemporal nerve (mandibular branch of trigeminal nerve, CN V)	Auricle Anterosuperior Anteromedial

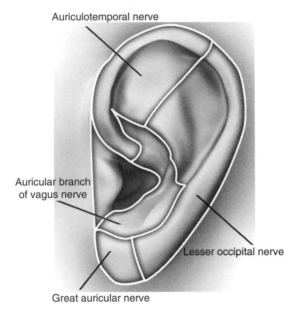

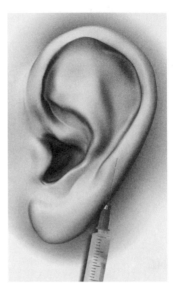

FIGURE 9.1 Nerve innervations of the ear.

FIGURE 9.2 Local nerve block—greater auricular and lesser occipital nerve block.

PROCEDURE PREPARATION

- Syringe (10 mL)
- Lidocaine 1% or bupivacaine 0.25%
- Needle—25- to 30-gauge

PROCEDURE

- Cleanse the area for infiltration with skin cleanser
- Fill the 10-mL syringe with either lidocaine or bupivacaine
- Attach the needle to the syringe

Local Nerve Branch Blocks

These are greater auricular and lesser occipital nerve branches (Figure 9.2).

- Insert needle at the posterior sulcus pointing to the superior pole following the curve of the auricle
- Gently aspirate and then inject 3 to 4 mL of anesthetic

Auriculotemporal Nerve Branch (Figure 9.3)

- Insert needle superior and anterior to the tragus
- Gently aspirate and then inject 2 to 4 mL of anesthetic

Ring Block/Regional Block (Figure 9.4)

- Insert the needle subcutaneously approximately 1-cm superior to the auricle in the direction just anterior to the tragus

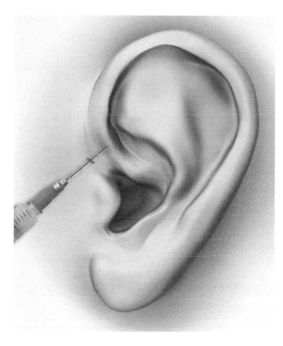

FIGURE 9.3 Local nerve block—auriculotemporal nerve block.

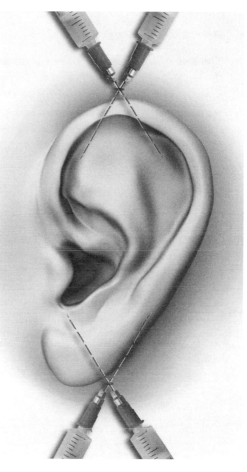

FIGURE 9.4 Ring-region nerve block of the ear.

- Gently aspirate and then inject 3 to 4 mL of anesthetic
- Remove the needle
- Insert the needle into the same place but direct it posteriorly
- Gently aspirate and then inject 3 to 4 mL of anesthetic
- Remove the needle
- Insert the needle inferior to the ear lobule
- Repeat the aforementioned steps injecting anteriorly and posteriorly

POSTPROCEDURE CONSIDERATIONS

- Pain with injection of anesthetic
- Consult ENT

COMPLICATIONS

- Possible cannulation of the superficial facial artery

Author's Pearls

The use of lidocaine with epinephrine has generally been contraindicated for the outer ear. However, recent literature suggests that the use of epinephrine does not block the circulation to this area of the ear and, therefore, does not cause necrosis. The decision to use epinephrine for local infiltration of the outer ear is at the clinician's discretion and should be based on the most up-to-date evidence-based practice. Epinephrine is also acceptable for regional block of the ear.

RESOURCES

Riviello, R. J., & Brown, N. A. (2010). Otolaryngologic procedures. In J. R. Roberts & J. Hedges (Eds.), *Clinical procedures in emergency medicine,* (5th ed., pp. 1195–1197). Philadelphia: Saunders Elsevier.

Rosh, A. J. (2009). Anesthesia, ear. Retrieved from http://emedicine.medscapre.com/article/82698-overview & http://emedicine.medscapre.com/article/82698-treatment

Overview of Wound Healing: Anatomy and Physiology

THERESA M. CAMPO

SKIN ANATOMY

Skin is a component of the integumentary system and is known as the cutaneous membrane. The cutaneous membrane consists of three major areas: cutaneous, subcutaneous, and deep fascia. It is a key component to our existence by providing protection, excretion, temperature regulation, sensory perception, and the synthesis of vitamin D. The skin also acts as a water barrier, specifically the stratum epithelial layer. Disruption in this layer can result in large water loss (i.e., burn victims).

Skin acts as a protective barrier to the external environment. It facilitates vasoconstriction and vasodilatation for temperature regulation and excretes salt, and water through perspiration. Nerve endings are encompassed to provide pain reception and the sensations of touch and pressure. Finally, skin is involved in the photosynthesis of vitamin D.

The dermal and epidermal layers comprise the cutaneous layer. The epidermis is the outermost layer and is made up of stratified squamous epithelial cells. There are two layers that are important to wound healing: the stratum germinativum, which continually makes new keratinocyts as old ones are shed (basal layer), and stratum corneum (horny or keratinized layer) layer that progressively moves up from the basal layer. The layers are very thin (0.2 mm thick) and difficult to differentiate from the dermal layer.

The dermis is the main component of the wound healing process. It is thicker and lies below the epidermis, and is made up primarily of connective tissue. The main cells of the dermis are fibroblasts, which are key in the facilitation of wound healing. They deposit fibrous proteins (elastin fibers and collagen), which give the wound its intrinsic strength. Blood vessels, nerves, and sebaceous and sudoriferous glands are contained within the loose connective tissue of this layer.

The layer lying beneath the dermis is the superficial fascia or subcutaneous layer. It is primarily composed of loose connective tissue and adipose tissue. These tissues provide insulation and protection to major blood vessels and underlying structures during trauma and significant temperature changes. Sensory nerves and major blood vessels pass through this layer.

The deepest layer is the deep fascial layer. It is composed of fibrous, thick, and dense tissue that supports the superficial layers of skin. This layer contains sensory nerve fibers, blood vessels, and lymphatics. The functions of this layer are to provide protection from the spread of infection, as well as to support and protect the underlying muscle and soft tissue structures. See Figure 10.1 for the layers of the skin.

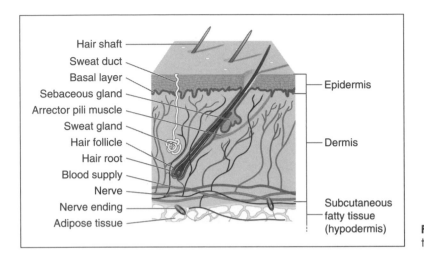

Hair shaft

Sweat duct

Basal layer

Sebaceous gland

Arrector pili muscle

Sweat gland

Hair follicle

Hair root

Blood supply

Nerve

Nerve ending

Adipose tissue

Epidermis

Dermis

Subcutaneous
fatty tissue
(hypodermis)

FIGURE 10.1 Layers of the skin.

PHASES OF WOUND HEALING

There are three main phases of wound healing. The components of the initial inflammatory phase are hemostatis and inflammation. The second phase is the proliferative phase and the final is the remodeling phase. There are many events occurring, separately and simultaneously. These phases begin at the onset of the wound and can continue for 1 to 2 years.

Hemostasis begins in minutes immediately after the injury via vasoconstriction, activation of the clotting cascade, and platelet aggregation. The platelets release thrombin and growth factors attracting fibroblasts and monocytes to the wound and the intrinsic clotting cascade is activated. This helps to limit the initial damage of the wound by ceasing bleeding and sealing the wound surface through retraction of the wound edges and clot formation.

The inflammatory phase is characterized by activation of the complement system, which causes increased vascular permeability, migration of cells into the wound and angiogenesis. Clinically this constitutes erythema, swelling, warmth, and pain. Chemoattractant agents bring the neutrophils and monocytes to the wound within 24 to 48 hours. The neutrophils clean the area by trapping and killing bacteria. The monocytes become tissue macrophages producing growth factors and cytokines to remove nonviable tissue and bacteria. Epidermal cells begin to migrate into the wound from surrounding tissue.

Neovascularization, fibroplasia, and epithelialization are the main components of the proliferative phase. Granulation occurs during this phase and the wound edges move closer together. A loose arrangement of collagen fibers begin to fill the wound as new capillaries begin to grow.

During the maturation phase, remodeling and wound contraction begin to occur. Wound contraction occurs as a result of myofibroblasts pulling collagen toward the cell body and epitheliazation is the migration of epithelial cells to resurface the wound. A more organized and stable form of collagen replaces the soft collagen. This increases the intrinsic tensile strength of the wound. This phase usually lasts about a year but can take 2 years to complete. Approximately 1 week after the wound occurs, the tensile strength is around 10% and at 1 year it can be 80%. Healed wounds never regain their original full tensile strength.

TYPES OF WOUND HEALING

Wound healing can occur by one of three ways: first intention, second intention, or third intention. First intention is when the wound is closed with sutures, staples, skin adhesive, or Steri-strips. Closure depends on time, contamination, and tissue devitalization. These are either clean lacerations or surgical incisions.

Second intention is when the wound is left open to heal on its own. This is a slower process than first intention and allows the wound to heal through granulation from the inside outward. These wounds can be caused by abscess, ulceration, puncture, or animal/human bites that are high risk of infection if closed primarily. These wounds can be grafted or revised at a later date when the risk of infection is considered minimal.

The final method of healing that is widely underutilized is a delayed primary closure. This is also known as third intention. Wounds that are significantly contaminated may be closed 4 to 5 days after occurrence to help reduce the risk of infection. This timeframe corresponds with the stages of wound healing when the risk of infection is significantly decreased. Delayed closures can occur weeks or months after the initial injury.

FACTORS COMPLICATING WOUND HEALING

Wound healing is a complex process that can be affected by numerous factors. Trauma, extent of wound, age, type of closure, alcoholism, diabetes, connective tissue disorders, medications, vitamin deficiencies, nutritional status, and circulation are all factors affecting wound healing. Consideration of underlying factors and prevention of further damage to the wound during any interventions are key to efficient wound healing.

WOUND CARE

Wound care before and after any procedure is crucial to wound healing. All wounds require cleansing with sterile normal saline. This can be completed through irrigation, scrubbing, and soaking. The method used will be dependent upon the type and extent of contamination of the wound. The use of hydrogen peroxide and povidone iodine are controversial and cause damage to viable tissue. Anytime these substances are used, they should be diluted. Whenever possible, commercially prepared skin cleanser should be used (i.e., chlorhexidine). Skin cleansers should also be used before any infiltration or invasive procedure to limit contamination with normal skin flora, dirt, and debris.

Author's Pearls

- *Wounds that are delayed in their healing or become worse have three general possibilities for the cause: retained foreign body, infection, and cancer.*
- *Pink or beefy red granulation tissue is a sign of proper wound healing **and** represents the proliferation phase.*

TYPES OF WOUNDS

There are six categories of wounds, which include abrasion, avulsion, combination, crush, laceration, and puncture. The characteristics and extent of the wound are dependent on the causative force. Please see Table 10.1 for the description of wounds in each of these categories and their causative force.

WOUND MANAGMENT

General care of all wounds presented throughout this book should be followed. Cleaning the skin with a skin cleanser (diluted povidone iodine or chlorhexidine) should be done before any injection procedure. Remember, the solution for pollution is dilution! Open wounds presenting to the provider should always be irrigated with normal saline before progressing with any procedure. It would be redundant to list this for each procedure involving an open wound. If a specific method of wound cleaning is necessary, then it will be noted in the respective chapters.

SPECIAL CONSIDERATIONS

Ring Removal

BACKGROUND

Any injury to the upper extremity can cause swelling to the finger(s). For this reason all rings should be removed before swelling begins. In cases where the edema has begun, the ring(s) can be removed using one of three techniques: lubricant, string technique, and ring cutter. Patients' rings not only have financial value but also

TABLE 10.1 Description of Wounds

Classification	Force	Wounds Characteristics	Example
Abrasion	Skin and object in opposite directions	Rough appearance with loss of epidermis and superficial dermis	"Road rash", "skinned knee"
Avulsion	Shearing Tensile force	Partial or complete loss of skin layers	Skin tear Flap of skin
Combination	Multiple forces cause wound: Crush, shear, tensile	Takes on numerous appearances depending on the force	Compression injury Explosions Motor vehicle crash
Crush	Compression of tissue against hard surface or bone	Devitalized tissue Ecchymosis surrounding wound	Rough, jagged wound edges
Laceration	Shear Compression Tensile	Clean, tidy Rough, jagged	Incision Knife injury Hitting head on solid object
Puncture	Tensile, compression	Depth of wound is greater than width Inability to visualize end of wound	Stepping on nail Bites

sentimental value. For these reasons attempts at removal with lubricant and/or string should be made before resorting to a ring cutter. Some metals are very strong, (i.e., Tungsten) and difficult to cut through and may lead to further injury of the digit (i.e., lacerations, edema).

PROCEDURAL PREPARATION

Lubricant
■ Gloves
■ Water-based lubricant (K-Y Jelly)
■ Gauze or paper towel

String Method
■ Gloves
■ Wide width Penrose drain or tourniquet
■ 20 inch length of string, umbilical tape, or 1/4 inch packing

Ring Cutter
■ Gloves
■ Manual or powered ring cutter

PROCEDURE

Lubricant
■ Liberally apply lubricant to the finger and rub around the ring
■ Turn the ring in a circular motion (one direction only)
■ Apply traction, moving the ring off the finger past the proximal interphalyngeal joint
■ Clean the finger with gauze or paper towel

String Method
If there is significant trauma to the finger or the patient is apprehensive and anxious, a digital block can be performed before beginning this procedure (see Chapter 5).

■ Take the penrose drain, or tourniquet, and wrap it around the finger distal to proximal
■ Allow it to stay in place for a few minutes (Figure 10.2)

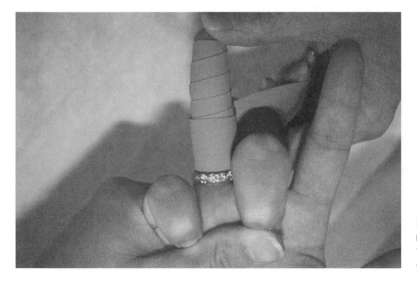

FIGURE 10.2 Ring removal—penrose-tourniquet application.

- Remove the penrose drain and pass the string material between the finger and ring
- Wrap the string from as close to the ring as possible distally on the finger
- Begin to unwrap the string from the proximal end (Figure 10.3), which will begin to move the ring off the finger

Ring Cutter
- Place the hook end of the cutter between the ring and finger (Figure 10.4)
- Allow the wheel to rest on the ring
- Begin turning the handle if the cutter is manual or start the power on the power cutter
- Once through the ring, attempt to spread the metal
- If the ends of the metal are too difficult to spread, another cut may be necessary

EDUCATIONAL POINTS
- Advise the patient that the ring can be repaired by a jeweler

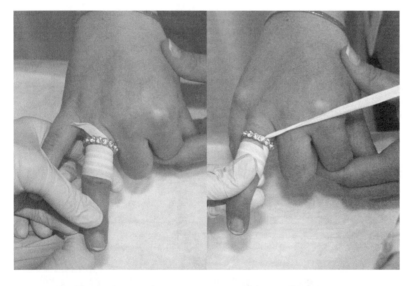

FIGURE 10.3 Ring removal—string application.

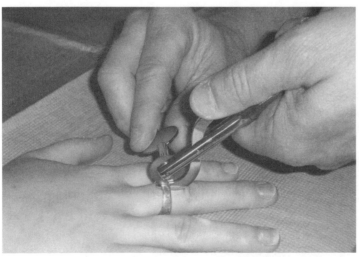

FIGURE 10.4 Ring removal—manual ring cutter.

> ## Author's Pearls
>
> - *Give reassurance and encouragement during the procedure*
> - *Ask if there are any inscriptions in the ring and try to avoid that area if possible*
> - *Manufactured ring cutters can either be manual, electrical, or battery operated (Figure 10.5)*

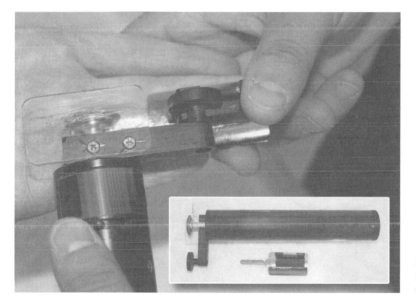

FIGURE 10.5 Ring removal—automatic ring cutter.

RESOURCES

Hollander, J. E. (2003). Patient and wound assessment: Basic concepts of the patient history and physical examination. In A. J. Singer & J. E. Hollander (Eds.), *Lacerations and acute wounds: An evidence-based guide* (pp. 9–12). Philadelphia: F. A. Davis Company.

Lammers, R. L. (2010). Principles of wound management. In J. R. Roberts & J. R. Hedges (Eds.), *Clinical procedures in emergency medicine* (5th ed., pp 563–575). Philadelphia: Saunders Elsevier.

Pieknik, R. (2006). Wounds. In *Suture and surgical hemostasis: A pocket guide.* (pp. 1–19). Philadelphia: Saunders.

Pieknik, R. (2006). Wound healing. In *Suture and surgical hemostasis: A pocket guide.* (pp. 20–41). Philadelphia: Saunders Elsevier.

Singer, A. J., & Clark, R. A. (2003). The biology of wound healing. In A. J. Singer & J. E. Hollander (Eds.), *Lacerations and acute wounds: An evidence-based guide* (pp. 1–8). Philadelphia: F. A. Davis Company.

Singer, A. J., & Clark, R. A. F. (1999). Cutaneous wound healing. *The New England Journal of Medicine, 341*(10), 738–746.

Trott, A. T. (2005). Anatomy of wound repair. In *Wounds and lacerations: Emergency care and closure* (3rd ed., pp. 13–18). Philadelphia: Mosby Elsevier.

Trott, A. T. (2005). Surface injury and wound healing. In *Wounds and lacerations: Emergency care and closure* (3rd ed., pp. 19–34). Philadelphia: Mosby Elsevier.

Trott, A. T. (2005). Wound care and the pediatric patient. In *Wounds and lacerations: Emergency care and closure* (3rd ed., pp. 35–48). Philadelphia: Mosby Elsevier.

Procedure for Managing Puncture Wounds

Theresa M. Campo

BACKGROUND

Puncture wounds can have a small or large opening depending upon the causative force and object (depth > width). Puncture wounds make it difficult to predict outcome because of the inability to visualize the end of the wound. The area of the body injured, level of contamination, and barriers between the offending object and the skin (i.e. shoes) can impact the interventions used and ultimate wound healing. Most importantly, the depth of penetration dictates innervation. Penetration into avascular structures such as bursae, tendons, and joint spaces allows organisms to proliferate. Some puncture wounds heal with minimal intervention; others become infected or have delayed healing regardless of the interventions and prophylaxis. Of note, 90% of puncture wounds to the foot involve stepping on a nail and 10–15% of these injuries become infected.

PATIENT PRESENTATION

- Pain
- Swelling
- Ecchymosis
- Open wound (can be as small as 1 mm)
- Bleeding

TREATMENT

Most puncture wounds have a smaller end than entrance of the wound, making cleaning and debriding difficult for the provider. Pressure irrigation of the puncture track can cause more damage by spreading contaminants and bacteria into surrounding tissue or spaces that cannot be visualized (e.g., tendon sheath of a puncture wound to the hand). Copious irrigation is the treatment method of choice. Forcible irrigation can also increase soft tissue swelling, lead to further tissue damage, and hinder healing.

Significantly contaminated puncture wounds can be treated by either performing a coring excision or incising the wound to convert it to a linear laceration. Determination for these techniques is based on the extent of the contamination, depth of the wound, presence of a foreign body, and the underlying tissue and structures. Plain films should be ordered when the possibility of a radiopaque FB is suspected; ultrasonography or exploration should occur with radiolucent foreign bodies.

SPECIAL CONSIDERATIONS

- Diabetics
- Immunocompromised patient
- Arterial or venous insufficiencies
- Anticoagulant therapy
- Steroids

PROCEDURE PREPARATION

- Absorbent pads
- Sterile normal saline solution
- Gauze
- Basin
- Splash guard or 16–18 gauge angio-catheter
- 35- or 65-mL syringe

If incising the area to remove contamination

- No. 11 or No. 15 scalpel
- Forceps

PROCEDURE

- Place the absorbent pad under the affected area
    - If the wound is on the hand, soak the area in normal saline and/or scrub the area. Otherwise the following procedure can be performed. Remember not to exert excessive pressure during irrigation.
- Adequate pressure needs to be 5–8 PSI and can be achieved with either the angio-catheter or splash shield and syringe
- Draw up the normal saline in the syringe
- Place the splash guard on the tip of the syringe
- Begin to irrigate the area
    - The rate of speed and the height of the stream will affect the amount of pressure on the tissue
- If the wound is contaminated, scrub the area to free the debris
- Irrigate to cleanse the area
- Apply antibiotic ointment and a dressing to the wound
    - For grossly contaminated areas: Incise the area to remove contamination (debridement)
- Cleanse the area
- Perform a local anesthesia (see Chapter 5)
- With the scalpel, extend the puncture wound (Figure 11.1)
- Debride the area of dirt, nonviable tissue, and foreign bodies
- Irrigate as described previously
- Apply topical antibiotic and dressing

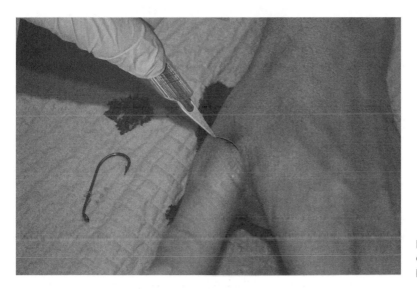

FIGURE 11.1 Incising a contaminated puncture wound.

POSTPROCEDURE CONSIDERATIONS

Antibiotic Prophylaxis

With contaminated wounds, antibiotic prophylaxis and tetanus prophylaxis should be considered. Puncture wounds occurring from stepping on a nail with a rubber-soled shoe should be treated with antibiotics that also address *Pseudomonas* infection, as this organism is harbored in rubber soled shoes (fluoroquinolone for adults and trimetoprim-sulfametoxazole for children).

Elevation

If the puncture wound is on an extremity, have the patient elevate the extremity to reduce the swelling or potential swelling resulting from the trauma. Reduction of swelling is key to promote tissue healing and to reduce pain.

Pain

Pain medication should be prescribed based on the patient's level of pain. Acetaminophen and nonsteroidal anti-inflammatory drugs are usually sufficient and well tolerated by the patient. Crutches can be used for a few days to reduce the discomfort of a puncture wound to the foot.

EDUCATIONAL POINTS

- Clean with soap and water
- Dressing changes daily and as needed
- Risk, benefits, and side effects of oral antibiotics, if prescribed
- Follow-up for wound evaluation 2 to 3 days postinjury

COMPLICATIONS

■ Infection, including cellulitis, deep space abscess, septic arthritis, and osteomyelitis, are a frequent complication of puncture wounds. Good wound hygiene at the time of injury and throughout the wound healing process, and close follow-up are key to prevention of infection.

■ Retained Foreign Body

AUTHOR'S PEARLS

■ *A combination of light irrigation and scrub can minimize contamination and the risk for infection*

■ *Puncture wounds occurring through rubber-soled shoes should be excised via a coring method*

■ *Pain is the most common symptom of infection*

■ *The greatest failure in treating a PW is the tendency to under-treat secondary to the benign appearance of the PW*

■ *All puncture wounds have a foreign body until proven otherwise*

RESOURCES

Lammers, R. (2003). Plantar puncture wounds. Basic concepts of the patient history: An physical examination. In A. J. Singer & J. E. Hollander (Eds.), *Lacerations and acute wounds: An evidence-based guide* (pp. 157–160). Philadelphia: F. A. Davis Company.

Lammers, R. L. (2010). Principles of wound management. In J. R. Roberts & J. R. Hedges (Eds.), *Clinical procedures in emergency medicine* (5th ed., pp. 565–566). Philadelphia: Saunders Elsevier.

Marx, J. A., Hockberger, R. S., & Walls, R. M. (2010). Forensic emergency medicine. In *Rosen's emergency medicine* (7th ed.). Retrieved from http://www.mdconsult.com/das/search/results/187068169-10?searchId=962524726&kw=puncture%20wound&bbSearchType=single&area=BookFast&set=1&DOCID=2084

Marx, J. A., Hockberger, R. S., & Walls, R. M. (2010). Wound management principles. *Rosen's emergency medicine* (7th ed.). Retrieved from http://www.mdconsult.com/book/player/book.do?method=display&type=bookPage&decorator=header&eid=4-u1.0-B978-0-323-05472-0..00056-6–s0320&uniq=187068169&isbn=978-0-323-05472-0&sid=962524726

Procedures for Removing a Soft Tissue Foreign Body

Theresa M. Campo

BACKGROUND

Foreign bodies (FBs) in the soft tissue can be of any material—organic material such as wood, thorns, and vegetative material, causing a rapid inflammatory response (usually infective); or inorganic material (glass, metal, plastic, and rubber), which usually do not cause a severe reaction. FBs are more common in children and occur most frequently on the extremities. The most commonly seen FBs are glass, wood, and metal. Your geographical region may influence the type and frequency of FB seen. For example, areas along the coast may see more fishhooks, wood splinters, and fish spines than the Midwest. Studies have shown more than one-third of soft tissue FBs are missed on initial examination.

Fishhooks can be a challenge to the provider. There are numerous types of hooks and the patient may not be astute to the type and size of the hook. Always ask the patient the type of hook (no barb, barbed with single or multiple barbs, or treble) (Figure 12.1). The technique for removal depends on the depth and type of hook that is embedded.

Ticks embed themselves in order to feed from their host. There are numerous types of ticks and they can carry bacteria, virus, toxins, spirochetes, Rickettsiae, and protozoa. Lyme disease, ehrlichiosis, Rocky Mountain spotted fever, and other illnesses can be caused by a prolonged tick bite.

PATIENT PRESENTATION

- Puncture wound with or without visible FB
- Pain
- Bleeding
- Discoloration (bruising, object)
- Swelling
- Nonhealing wound
- Granuloma formation
- Cellulitis
- Abscess formation

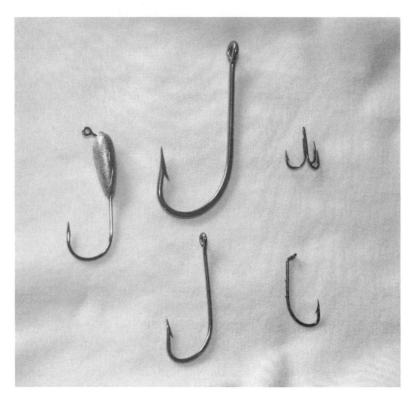

FIGURE 12.1 Type of fishhooks.

TREATMENT

Treatment is based on the location, depth, timing, and type of FB. Organic FBs do not show on plain radiographs. They are better visualized with ultrasound (US). CT scan can also be used to visualize FBs with a higher sensitivity than plain radiographs. The overall sensitivity is 95%, specifically 100% for metal, 75% for glass, and 7% for wood. It is more expensive than plain radiographs and should be used when a FB is suspected and not found on x-ray or ultrasound. Metal and glass can be well visualized on plain radiographs except when hidden by bone or if very small (usually <5 mm). Multiple views on plain x-ray are needed to detect FBs. Plastic materials may show on plain radiographs but are better seen with ultrasound.

Plain radiographs and ultrasound are beneficial and cost effective. Radiographs allow for visualization and estimation of depth. Ultrasound can be used for guided removal of elusive and organic FBs and is mainstream for detecting radiolucent FBs (greater than 90% sensitivity) such as wood and rubber when used properly.

There are various methods for FB removal, and they are based on the location, type, and depth of the FB. The possible positions of FBs in regard to soft tissue are superficial horizontal, vertical, subungual, and elusive. There are multiple methods for fishhook removal, which will also be discussed in this chapter.

Superficial horizontal FBs sit in the dermal and epidermal layer of the skin along the horizontal axis. You can see and palpate the FB, and it can be removed by excision. The vertical FB is perpendicular to the skin surface with only a very small surface, if any, exposed. This FB is difficult to remove and can be very deep. Incision and coring is used to remove this FB. The subungual FB is located beneath the nail plate. Cutting the nail in a "V" shape and removing the splinter is the most common method of removal. Performing a digital block and elevating the nail for removal is another option. Elusive FBs usually require referral for guided removal with either fluoroscopy or ultrasound. Plain radiographs can assist with placement and depth of the FB. However, the object may become displaced when an incision is made, making removal more complicated and causing more trauma to the tissue.

Obtaining the location, mechanism, timing, material of the FB, occupation, tetanus status, history of diabetes or immunosuppression, and hand dominance (if upper extremity is involved) are key features of the history. Assessment of contamination, location of FB, surrounding structural function (nerve, tendon, muscle, etc.) are imperative to ensure that the provider properly identifies and provides proper treatment of the patient. If the patient states that he or she feels an FB, you must exhaust all measures to confirm whether there is an FB. A missed FB can lead to infections, including osteomyelitis deep space abscess, and granuloma formation.

CONTRAINDICATIONS AND RELATIVE CONTRAINDICATIONS

- Deep elusive FBs
- Inability to obtain and maintain hemostasis for complete evaluation and removal
- Poor cosmetic outcome

SPECIAL CONSIDERATIONS

- Diabetics
- Immunocompromised
- Anticoagulant therapy

PROCEDURE PREPARATION

Foreign Body

SUPERFICIAL HORIZONTAL, VERTICAL, AND SUBUNGUAL
- Skin cleanser
- Absorbant pad
- Gloves
- Topical or injectable anesthetic
  - Small, superficial, and/or callused skin may not require any anesthetic
- No. 11 or No. 15 scalpel
- Splinter or fine forceps
- Small scissors
- Hemostat
- Normal saline for irrigation
- 35–65 mL syringe (for irrigation)
- 16–18 gauge angiocath or splash guard
- Skin cleanser scrub
- Dressing material
- Antibiotic ointment

ELUSIVE

Removal should not be attempted if the object cannot be visualized. Referral is recommended for these patients.

Fishhook

RETROGRADE
- Gloves
- Normal saline for irrigation
- Skin cleanser

STRING YANK
- Gloves
- Normal saline for irrigation
- Skin cleanser
- String (thick suture material or umbilical tape)

NEEDLE COVER
- Gloves
- Normal saline for irrigation
- Skin cleanser
- Injectable anesthetic
- Large-gauge needle (18 gauge or larger)

ADVANCE AND CUT
- Gloves
- Normal saline for irrigation
- Skin cleanser
- Injectable anesthetic
- Needle driver, hemostat, or pliers

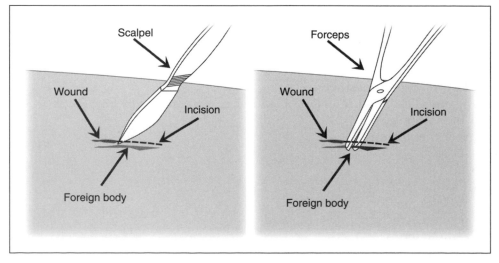

FIGURE 12.2 Superficial horizontal FB removal technique.

PROCEDURE

Foreign Body

SUPERFICIAL HORIZONTAL (FIGURE 12.2)

■ Cleanse the skin
■ Use topical or local anesthetic
  ■ The type of anesthetic is determined by size, location, and depth of the FB and patient tolerance
■ Make an incision along the FB. Incise the entire length to ensure full removal
■ Apply gentle pressure to one end of the FB while lifting the opposite side
■ Grab the FB with forceps
■ Irrigate with copious amount of normal saline
■ Scrub the area to loosen debris and contamination, if necessary
■ Apply dry sterile dressing with antibiotic ointment

VERTICAL (FIGURE 12.3)

■ Cleanse the skin
■ Perform local anesthetic
■ Make an incision over the FB
■ Secure the FB, if possible, with the forceps
■ Incise around the FB (coring)

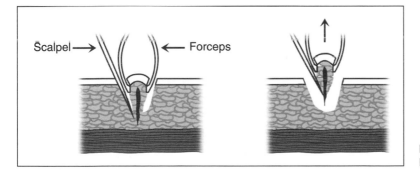

FIGURE 12.3 Vertical FB removal technique.

■ Remove the entire section
■ Irrigate with copious amount of normal saline
■ Scrub the area to loosen debris and contamination, if necessary
■ Apply dry sterile dressing with antibiotic ointment

SUBUNGUAL (FIGURE 12.4)

■ Cleanse the area
■ Perform a digital block
■ With either the scalpel or a small scissors cut a "V" shape from the distal nail
  ■ The point of the "V" should go to the proximal end of the FB
  ■ Be careful not to cut or cause undue trauma to the nail bed
■ Remove the piece of nail with either the forceps or hemostat

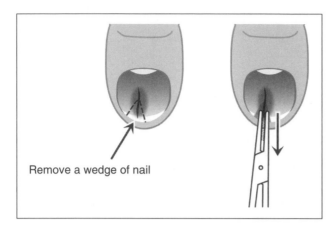

Remove a wedge of nail

FIGURE 12.4 Removal of a subungual FB.

- Grasp the FB with the splinter forceps and remove by gently pulling
- Irrigate with copious amount of normal saline
- Scrub the area to loosen debris and contamination if necessary
- Apply dry sterile dressing with antibiotic ointment

Fishhook

Key to successful removal of fishhooks is disengaging the barb from the tissue.

RETROGRADE (FIGURE 12.5)
This technique should be used for hooks that are barbless and superficial. It can be attempted if the hook is small and barbed.

- Apply downward pressure to the base or shank of the hook
- Gently rotate to disengage the barb
- Begin to back out the hook
  - Any resistance, stop the procedure and use another method

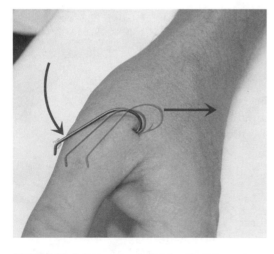

FIGURE 12.5 Retrograde fishhook removal technique.

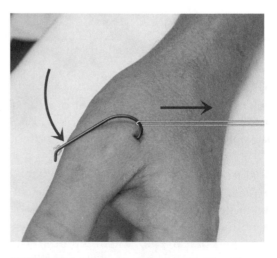

FIGURE 12.6 String-yank fishhook removal technique.

- Irrigate with copious amount of normal saline
- Scrub the area to loosen debris and contamination, if necessary
- Apply dry sterile dressing with antibiotic ointment

STRING YANK (FIGURE 12.6)

This technique is best for small to medium fishhooks. Successful removal is best on fixed body parts.

- Cleanse the area
- Topical or local anesthetic may be needed based on the patient tolerance
- Wrap the string around the center of the fishhook
- Hold the ends tight
- Rest the affected area on the table
- Apply downward pressure to the base or shank of the hook
- Push the distal end of the hook (the eye) against the skin while pulling on the string
- Irrigate with copious amount of normal saline
- Scrub the area to loosen debris and contamination, if necessary
- Apply dry sterile dressing with antibiotic ointment

NEEDLE COVER (FIGURE 12.7)

This technique can be used for any size fishhook with a single barb.

- Cleanse the area
- Perform local anesthesia
- Line up the large-gauge needle with the bevel facing the hook
- Advance the needle through the opening and follow the hook
- Push the hook forward and down slightly
    - You may have to slightly rotate the fishhook to help disengage the tissue

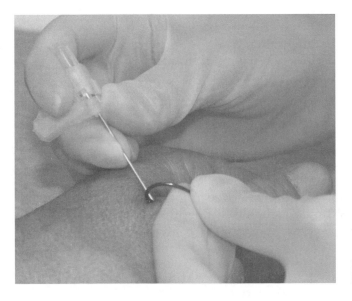

FIGURE 12.7 Needle cover fishhook removal technique.

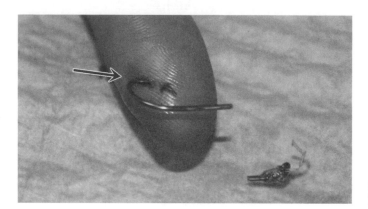

FIGURE 12.8 Advance and cut fishhook removal technique.

- Then begin to pull the hook out with the bevel of needle over the barb
- Irrigate with copious amount of normal saline
- Scrub the area to loosen debris and contamination, if necessary
- Apply dry sterile dressing with antibiotic ointment

ADVANCE AND CUT (FIGURE 12.8)
This technique can be used for any size hook with a single or multiple barbs.

Single Barb
- Cleanse the area
- Perform local anesthesic
- Push the point of the fishhook through the skin where it was tenting
  - If unable to push through the skin, make a small incision
- Grab and secure the point of the hook with a needle driver or hemostat
- Cut the point of the hook below the barb with wire cutters or other available cutting tools
- Grasp the proximal end of the hook (the eye) and back out the hook
- Irrigate with copious amount of normal saline
- Scrub the area to loosen debris and contamination, if necessary
- Apply dry sterile dressing with antibiotic ointment

Multiple Barb
- Follow the aforementioned procedure, but cut the eye of the hook and pull the hook by the point (barb end)

Postprocedure Considerations

- Copious irrigation is needed after the FB is removed
- Marine spines (sting ray, lion fish, and sea urchin) carry slime and calcareous material and are associated with granuloma formation—coverage for Vibrio infection should be considered

- A nail through a rubber-soled shoe should be covered for Pseudomonas infection with ciprofloxacin or another fluoroquinolone. Children should receive trimethoprim–sulfamethoxazole.

Tick Removal

There are over-the-counter tick removal devices (TRIX, Tick key, Sawyer tick pliers, etc.). Do not apply any products to the tick to attempt to kill or "stun" the tick. This may cause the tick to regurgitate and spread infection.

- Don gloves. Ticks can pass infection with direct contact, not just bites
- With fine-tipped forceps grasp the tick as close to the skin as possible
- Apply even traction while pulling upward until the tick is removed
  - Do not twist, crush, or jerk when removing
  - Inspect for and remove any retained mouth or body parts
- Cleanse the area with soap and water

EDUCATIONAL POINTS

- Complete removal of the FB and irrigation is essential
- Antibiotic prophylaxis and close follow-up for grossly contaminated wounds and for patients with comorbidity are recommended
- Have the patient regularly clean the wound with soap and water and apply antibiotic ointment

COMPLICATIONS

- Infection
- Retained foreign body
- Further injury
  - Surrounding tissue during removal
  - Neurovascular

AUTHOR'S PEARLS

- *Education and counseling go a long way with patients with tick bites as most patients and parents are very anxious about the risk of Lyme disease and other illnesses. There are limited studies with regard to antibiotic prophylaxis and the use of a one-time dose of doxycycline. The studies that have been done have shown that the incidence of transmission is low and the use of antibiotic prophylaxis inconclusive. Testing for Lyme disease should not be done immediately after the tick bite and/or after tick removal due to the high incidence of false results.*
- *Always use the proper type and amount of anesthesia before FB exploration.*
- *The use of a tourniquet for hemostasis will aid in visualization and removal of FBs*

RESOURCES

Bass, A. M., & Levis, J. T. (2010). Foreign body removal, wound. Retrieved from http:// emedicine.medscape.com/article/1508207-overview & http://emedicine.medscape.com/ article/1508207-treatment

Chan, C., & Salam, G. A. (2003). Splinter removal. *American Family Physician, 67*(12), 2557–2562.

Consoli, R. J. (2007). Emergency medicine. In R. E. Rakel (Ed.), *Textbook of family medicine* (7th ed.). Philadelphia: Saunders Elsevier. Retrieved from http://www.mdconsult. com/das/book/body/187280795-6/963092363/1481/466.html#4-u1.0-B978-1-4160-2467-5..50042-7–cesec45_2366

Edlow, J. A. (2009). Tick-borne diseases, Lyme. Retrieved from http://emedicine.medscape.com/ article/1413603-overview & http://emedicine.medscape.com/article/1413603-treatment

Halaas, G. W. (2007). Management of foreign bodies in the skin. *Amer ican Family Physician, 76*(5), Retrieved from http://www.mdconsult.com/das/article/body/187280795-4/jorg= journal&source=MI&sp=19952104&sid=963088564/N/607270/1.html?issn=0002-838X

Lammers, R. (2003). Foreign bodies in wounds. In A. J. Singer & J. E. Hollander (Eds.), *Lacerations and acute wounds: An evidence-based guide* (pp. 147–156). Philadelphia: F. A. Davis Company.

Otten, E. J., & Mohler, D. G. (2007). Hunting and other weapon injuries. In P. S. Auerbach (Ed.), *Wilderness medicine* (5th ed.). Philadelphia: Mosby Elsevier. Retrieved from http:// www.mdconsult.com/das/book/body/187280795-6/963092363/1483/198.html#4-u1.0-B978-0-323-03228-5..50027-6–cesec16_1268

Shiels, W. E. (2007). Soft tissue foreign bodies: Sonographic diagnosis and therapeutic management. *Ultrasound Clinics, 2*(4), Retrieved from http://www.mdconsult.com/das/article/ body/187280795-4/jorg=journal&source=&sp=20606707&sid=963088564/N/638044/1. html?issn=1556-858X

Stone, D. B., & Levine, M. R. (2010). Foreign body removal. In J. R. Roberts & J. R. Hedges (Eds.), *Clinical procedures in emergency medicine* (5th ed., pp. 634–648). Philadelphia: Saunders Elsevier.

Thommasen, H. V. (2005). The occasional removal of an embedded fish hook. *Canadian Journal of Rural Medicine, 10*(4), 254–259.

Managing Animal and Human Bites

THERESA M. CAMPO

BACKGROUND

Animal bites can occur at any age and for many reasons. Animal bites in children usually occur from "roughhousing" with a pet or bothering an animal when it does not want to be disturbed. Bites in adults usually occur while attempting to break up fighting dogs or attempting to assist a distressed animal. Any unprovoked attack should be considered suspicious for rabies. Patients should be covered for rabies in any suspicious bite where the offending animal cannot be located and quarantined/tested. The patient's tetanus immunization status should be assessed and vaccination with either tetanus toxoid, or tetanus with diphtheria and pertussis should be administered. The tetanus with diphtheria and pertussis is based on the patient's age. Please refer to the new guidelines.

Dog bites most frequently occur in children 10 years old or younger and occur on the face, neck, and/or head and represent 80–90% of bites presenting to the emergency department. Bites to adults usually occur on the hands or arms from attempting to break up dogs that are fighting. Dog bites become infected less than 15% of the time. The teeth of dogs are round and large and tend to cause more crushing injuries than cats and can generate 200–450 PSI and can crush sheet metal. Wound care, as well as the possibility for soft tissue injury, bone fracture, and foreign bodies should always be considered.

Cat bites are less frequent and are at greater risk of becoming infected. The bite of a cat tends to leave deeper puncture wounds but are smaller in size than that of a dog. The teeth of cats are sharp and pointed and tend to "inoculate" bacteria deep into the tissue. When infection occurs, it is usually more rapid than a dog bite and can include muscle, bone, and, most frequently, tendons (especially in the hands).

Human bites are the least frequently occurring but have a high rate of infection due to the polymicrobial nature of the human mouth. There are numerous organisms that can be found in our mouths at any given time. These bites can occur from altercations, assaults, sexual activity, seizures, and during medical and dental procedures (Figure 13.1). Bites can be either intentional (true bite) or unintentional (closed fist).

A true bite can occur from the action of being bitten unintentionally when two people collide and the tooth of one person is pushed into the skin of another. Any open wound on the dorsal aspect of the hand, especially over the fourth or fifth metacarpalphalyngeal (MP) joint, is considered to be a bite when it occurs with a closed hand or fist. Most patients will deny this mechanism to avoid "getting into trouble." However, it is important to discuss the increased risk of infection with

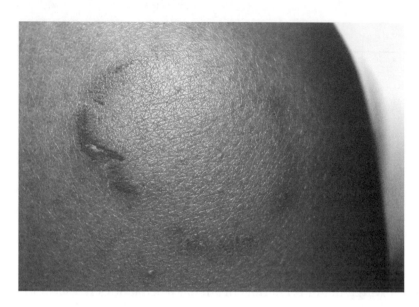

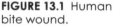

FIGURE 13.1 Human bite wound.

these injuries and reassure patients that they will not be penalized for their honesty. It is also very important to document the discussion on the patient's chart. It is of extreme importance to evaluate the joints for range of motion (ROM) in order to uncover a tendon and/or joint injury. Furthermore, these wounds may need to be extended in order to properly visualize the extent of the wound.

Another important consideration with human bites is the risk of transmission of hepatitis, human immunodeficiency virus (HIV), syphilis, and other communicable diseases. Whenever possible, the patient and the person causing the bite, regardless of method, should be tested.

PATIENT PRESENTATION

Patients with either human or animal bites can present with varying degrees of severity and injuries.

- Pain
- Swelling
- Abrasion
- Ecchymosis
- Laceration
- Puncture wound
- Avulsion or partial avulsion
- Crushing injury
- Redness
- Drainage

TREATMENT

The goals of treatment are hemostasis, minimizing the risk of infection, reducing swelling, debridement of devitalized tissue, and improving cosmetic outcome. History should include the time of the injury, circumstances leading up to the attack, and past medical history of diabetes, immunosuppression, chemotherapeutics, and the immunization status of the patient and animal or human attacker. Radiographs should be ordered to rule out fracture and/or foreign body. Injuries to the hand, involving a punch injury, should always be assessed for full range of motion, tendon and joint function, and strength in all digits. Copious irrigation and debridement should also be performed and referred to a hand specialist for close follow-up.

Minor injuries can be treated with direct pressure, irrigation/washing, topical antibiotic and ice, and elevation for swelling. Major bites can be deep, extensive, and involve the head, face, hands, and extremities. The severity and type of injury stipulates the treatment required. Facial wounds should be closed by primary intention, and should be given antibiotics and close follow-up. Recommended antibiotics and common organisms from dog, cat, and human bites can be viewed in Table 13.1.

CONTRAINDICATIONS AND RELATIVE CONTRAINDICATIONS

Age of the Wound

- Wounds that are older than 8 hours should be left open to heal by second intention. The older the wound, the higher the risk for developing infection
  - Dog bites to the face can be sutured up to 12 hours after the bite. Some literature even recommends up to 24 hours as long as antibiotic prophylaxis and close follow-up are done
  - Delay in evaluation and treatment leads to increased rates of infection

Cause of the Wound

- Human and cat bites should not be closed unless they are very large due to the risk of infection. Cat bites should not be closed when they involve the hand

History of Diabetes, Immunosuppression, and HIV

- Patients with diabetes, immunosuppression, and HIV should have close follow-up. The wounds should remain open and heal by second intent unless gaping

PROCEDURAL PREPARATION

- Absorbent pad
- Normal saline for irrigation
- 35–65 mL syringe
- Splash shield or 16–18 gauge angio-catheter
- Surgical scrub
- 4 × 4 gauze
- Topical antibiotic

Any bite to the hand or any human or cat bite should not be closed by first intention. Bites to the hand tend to have a higher infection rate (up to 28%) due to the number of enclosed compartments, nerves, tendons, joints and fascial planes. Closure by second intention may be the best option due to the higher infection rate. Refer Chapter 14 for closure techniques.

TABLE 13.1 Common Organisms and Antibiotic Treatment for Dog, Cat, and Human Bites

Bite	Organism(s)	First-line Antibiotic	Alternative
Dog	**Aerobic** ■ *Pasteurella multocida* ■ *Staphylococcus aureus* ■ *Streptococcus* species **Anaerobic** ■ *Cornebacterium* species ■ *Eikenella corrodans* ■ *Capnocytphaga canimorsus*	Prophylaxis—3 to 5 days Infection—10 days ■ Amoxicillin-clavulonate	Doxycycline ■ 8 years old ■ Pregnancy ■ Penicillin allergy **Adults** ■ Clindamycin and fluoroquinolone **Children** ■ Clindamycin and trimethoprim-sulfamethoxazole
Cat	**Aerobic** ■ *Pasteurella multocida* ■ *Streptococcus* species (inc. *S. pyogenes*) ■ *Staphylococcus aureus* ■ *Moraxella cataralis* **Anaerobic** ■ Fusobacterium ■ *Bacteroids fragilis* ■ Porphyromonas ■ *Capnocytophaga canimorsus*	Prophylaxis—3 to 5 days Infection—10 days ■ Amoxicillin-clavulonate Do not use cephalexin	Doxycycline ■ 8 years old ■ Pregnancy ■ Penicillin allergy **Adults** ■ Clindamycin and fluoroquinolone **Children** ■ Clindamycin and trimethoprim-sulfamethoxazole
Human	**Aerobic** ■ *Eikenella corrodans* ■ Alpha and beta hemolytic streptococcus ■ *Staphylococcus aureus* and *S. epidermidis* ■ *Corynebacterium* species **Anaerobic** ■ *Peptostreptylococcus* species ■ *Bacteroid fragilis* and nonfragilis ■ Fusobacterium ■ Veillonella	Prophylaxis—3 to 5 days Infection—10 days ■ Amoxicillin-clavulonate ■ Ampicillin/sulbactam	Clindamycin and trimethoprim-sulfamethoxazole ■ Penicillin allergy ■ Children ■ Pregnancy

PROCEDURE

■ Place the absorbent pad under the effected area
■ Pour the normal saline into the basin
■ Draw up the saline with the syringe
■ Place the splash shield or catheter on the end of the syringe. (Do not use high pressure irrigation with bites to the hands.)

- Irrigate the area
- Use a surgical scrub to free any debris
- Dry completely
- Apply topical antibiotic
- Dress the wound

POSTPROCEDURE CONSIDERATIONS

Infection

If the wounds are 8 hours and older, contaminated, involve bone, joint or tendon, or the patient has diabetes or immunosuppression, then it is best to leave them open for secondary healing. Broad spectrum antibiotics can be prescribed for approximately 5 days to help prevent infection. Groin injuries should also be considered for antibiotic prophylaxis.

Pain

Pain medication should be prescribed based upon the severity of the injury and pain tolerance. Elevation and ice can help reduce the swelling and pain.

Rabies Prophylaxis

Rabies prophylaxis should be initiated with any suspicious animal bite (i.e., strays). The patient should receive rabies immunoglobin 20 IU/kg. Inject up to 50% around the wound(s) and the remainder via intramuscular (IM) injection. The patient will need to receive the rabies vaccine (Imovax, RabAvert) on the day of the injury, day 0, and on days 3, 7, 14, and 28. The dose is standard at 1 mL IM in the deltoid.

EDUCATIONAL POINTS

- Dressings should remain in place for 24 hours
- Clean with soap and water
- Antibiotic ointment should be applied
- Apply topical antibiotics to facial wounds frequently (every couple of hours) to avoid crusting and scar

COMPLICATIONS

- Infection is always a consideration with bite wounds
  - Dogs have the lowest incidence of infection
    - Parallel nonbite wound infection rates
  - Cat bites have the highest infection rate of 60% to 80% due to the shape and structure of the teeth
  - Facial wounds
    - Excellent blood supply
    - Low risk for infection, even if closed primarily
    - Risk of superinfection must be discussed with the patient prior to closure
    - Generally, the better the vascular supply and the easier the wound is to clean (i.e., laceration vs. puncture), the lower the risk of infection
- Early intervention, cleaning of the wounds, and close follow-up can help prevent these infections

Author's Pearls

■ *If the wound is gaping, you can loosely close the wounds so that it can drain and easily be opened if needed*

■ *Rapid onset of infection, usually within 12–24 hours, tends to be caused by* Pasteurella multocida *where as most other infections present 48–72 hours after the injury*

■ *Bites to the hands, from any source, demands the use of antibiotics and no closure*

■ *First generation antibiotics are not as effective as Amoxicillin-clavulonate due to resistance by* Eikenella corrodans *and anaerobic organisms*

RESOURCES

Barrett, J., & McNamara, R. M. (2010, April 8). Bites, human. Retrieved from http://emedicine.medscape.com/article/768978-overview & http://emedicine.medscape.com/article/768978-treatment

Dire, D. J. (2003). Animal bites. In A. J. Singer & J. E. Hollander (Eds.), *Lacerations and acute wounds: An evidence-based guide* (pp. 133–146). Philadelphia: F. A. Davis Company.

Freer, L. (2007). Bites and injuries inflicted by wild and domestic animals. In P. S. Auerbach (Ed.). *Wilderness medicine* (5th ed.). Philadelphia: Mosby Elsevier. Retrieved from http://www.mdconsult.com/das/book/body/187280795-8/0/1483/457.html?tocnode=54236968&fromURL=457.html#4-u1.0-B978-0-323-03228-5..50056-2_2767

Habif, T. P. (2009). Animal and human bites. In *Clinical dermatology: A color guide to diagnosis and treatment* (5th ed.). Retrieved from http://www.mdconsult.com/book/player/book.do?method=display&type=bookPage&decorator=header&eid=4-u1.0-B978-0-7234-3541-9..00024-9–s0735&uniq=187280795&isbn=978-0-7234-3541-9&sid=963112235#lpState=open&lpTab=contentsTab&content=4-u1.0-B978-0-7234-3541-9..00024-9-s0735%3Bfrom%3Dtoc%3Btype%3DbookPage%3Bisbn%3D978-0-7234-3541-9

Lee, C. K., & Hansen, S. L. (2009). Management of acute wounds. *Surgical clinics of North America, 89*(3), 659-676.

Oehler, R. L., Velez, A. P., Mizrachi, M., Lamarche, J., & Gompf, S. (2009). Bite related and septic syndromes caused by dogs and cats. *Lancet, 9,* 439–447.

Perkins, A., & Harris, N. S. (2009, June 25). Bites, animal. Retrieved from http://emedicine.medscape.com/article/768875-overview & http://emedicine.medscape.com/article/768875-treatment

Prescutti, R. J. (2001). Prevention and treatment of dog bites. *American Family Physicians, 63,* 1567–1574.

Shoemaker, D. M., Jiang, P. P., Williamson, H., & Roland, W. E. (2007). Infectious disease: Bite infections. In R. E. Rakel (Ed.), *Textbook of family medicine* (7th ed.). Philadelphia: Saunders Elsevier. Retrieved from http://www.mdconsult.com/das/book/body/187280795-12/0/1481/241.html#4-u1.0-B978-1-4160-2467-5..50024-5–cesec111

Rhoads, J. (2009). Managing bites and stings. *The Nurse Practitioner, 34*(8), 37–43.

Weber, E. J., & West, H. H. (2010). Mammalian bites. In *Rosen's emergency medicine* (7th ed.). Retrieved from http://www.mdconsult.com/book/player/book.do?method=display&type=bookPage&decorator=header&eid=4-u1.0-B978-0-323-05472-0..00058-X&displayedEid=4-u1.0-B978-0-323-05472-0..00058-X–s0010&uniq=187280795&isbn=978-0-323-05472-0&sid=963109534

Wound Closure Procedures

Theresa M. Campo

BACKGROUND

The goal of wound healing through primary intent is to facilitate decreased healing time, reduce infection, and minimize scarring. This can be achieved through rapid assessment and interventions to minimize contamination, debriding devitalized tissue, obtaining hemostasis, removal of foreign body, and approximating tissue edges. It is imperative to make an accurate and thorough assessment of not only the wound, but also of the circumstances that led to the wound (mechanism and time). It is also important to assess for past medical history including diabetes, allergies to anesthetics, neurological and motor function, presence or suspicion of foreign body, and underlying structural damage (tendon, vessel, joint capsule, and nerve).

Delay in wound healing can have multifaceted consequences. The mechanism of the injury alone can put the patient at risk for infection and complication (i.e., crush, foreign body, etc.). Medical conditions and medications also play a role in wound healing. Patients with diabetes, immunosuppression, obesity, malnutrition, tobacco use, older age, and steroid usage are at greater risk for infections and delayed wound healing. It is important to help the patient to manage these risk factors whenever possible.

PATIENT PRESENTATION

- Pain
- Bleeding
- Open wound(s)
- Decreased or loss of sensation or function
- Anxiety

TREATMENT

Treatment begins with a thorough history including mechanism, time of incident, medications, medication allergies, and immunization status (tetanus). Once the history is complete, do a careful examination of the wound and surrounding areas to ensure that there are no hidden foreign bodies or other injuries. If a foreign body is suspected, further studies should be ordered (plain radiograph, ultrasound, etc.). Regardless of the size of the wound, the patient will experience pain and should be anesthetized before wound cleansing and exploration.

The skin should be cleansed, the area anesthetized then irrigated with moderate pressure (5–8 PSI with normal saline irrigation), and/or gently scrubbed. Once this has been completed, the wound should be probed for debris, foreign body, and devitalized tissue. The type of closure will depend upon the type of wound, location, time since injury, contamination and depth. Suture, staple, skin adhesive, and tape closures will be discussed in this chapter. Each method has its advantages and disadvantages, which will be discussed at the beginning of each procedure type. Because of wound contraction during the healing phase, eversion is of paramount importance in all closures.

CONTRAINDICATIONS AND RELATIVE CONTRAINDICATIONS

- Grossly contaminated wounds
- Cause of the wound(s)
  - Puncture wound
  - Human and animal bite (depending upon source and location)
- Delay in seeking treatment
  - Face and scalp—up to 24 hours
  - Hands and feet—<6 hours

SPECIAL CONSIDERATIONS

- Diabetes
- Immunosuppression
- Tobacco use
- Steroids
- Chemo- and radiation therapies
- Malnutrition

PROCEDURE PREPARATION

- Nonsterile gloves
- Absorbable pad
- 4 × 4 gauze
- Skin cleanser
- Topical anesthetic
- Injectable anesthetic
- Normal saline for irrigation
- 20- to 30-mL syringe
- Splash guard
- Surgical scrub
- Nonadherent gauze
- Topical antibiotic

Suture

- Sterile gloves
- Suture kit (needle holder, toothed forceps, suture scissors, sterile drapes, basin and cups for cleanser, and normal saline)
- Suture material
  - Subcuticular and subcutaneous—absorbable (vicryl, chromic)

■ Percutaneous—nonabsorbable (nylon, polypropylene)
■ Face—thinner material (6–0)
■ Extremities, torso, and scalp (3–0 to 5–0)

Staple

■ Sterile gloves
■ Suture kit (needle holder, toothed forceps, suture scissors, sterile drapes, basin and cups for cleanser, and normal saline)
■ Staple gun

Skin Adhesive

■ Sterile pack 4 × 4 gauze
■ Skin adhesive (Cyanoacrylate glue–Dermabond©, Indermill©)
■ Skin tape (Steri-strips, butterflies)

Tape

■ Benzoin
■ Cotton-tipped applicators
■ Skin tape (1/4 inch, 1/2 inch)

PROCEDURE

Suture

This is a great method of wound closure offers preciseness, wound edge approximation, and tensile strength. The disadvantages of sutures are the need for injectable
anesthetic, removal of the sutures, tissue reactivity (especially with absorbable sutures),
increased cost, and increased time to perform the procedure. There is also a great
expectation by the patient or parents for a "perfect closure" and no scar formation.

■ Put on nonsterile gloves
■ Cleanse the skin
■ Apply topical anesthetic
  ■ Children, especially faces
■ Perform local, digital, or regional block based on the location and size of the wound (see Chapter 5)
■ While the anesthetic is taking effect, open the suture kit and place the equipment needed onto your sterile field
■ Put on sterile gloves
■ Draw up the normal saline for irrigation in the large syringe
■ Attach the splash guard
■ Irrigate the wound with moderate pressure 5–8 PSI which can be achieved using a 35–65 mL syringe and either a splash shield or 16–18 gauge angio-catheter
  ■ Use a gentle scrub for the eyebrow and around the eye as pressure irrigation can cause further damage to this sensitive area
■ Gently scrub the area if there is debris and contamination that was not removed with irrigation
■ Place the fenestrated sterile drape over the wound

- Probe and visualize the wound for debris, contamination and devitalized tissue and remove
- Open the suture material
- Hold the needle holder in your dominant hand with the thumb in one hole and the ring finger in the other (Figure 14.1)
- Using your index finger to support the needle holder, open the locking mechanism
- Grab the suture needle at the 1/3 junction of the proximal and mid section
  - The needle holder should be perpendicular to the needle (Figure 14.2)
- Secure the locking mechanism
- Remove the fingers from the holes and hold the needle holder in the palm of your hand
- Put the forceps in your nondominant hand between the thumb and index fingers (Figure 14.3)
- Use the forceps to gently evert the wound edge
- Insert the needle at 90° to the skin (Figure 14.4) and press the needle through the skin and out the center of the wound. This angle ensures proper skin edge eversion
  - Supinate your hand to give the proper motion and direction through the skin
- Release the needle

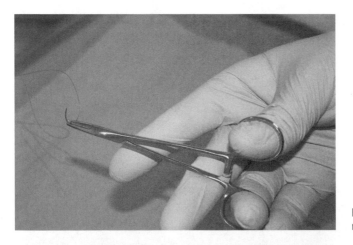

FIGURE 14.1 Proper way to hold a needle holder.

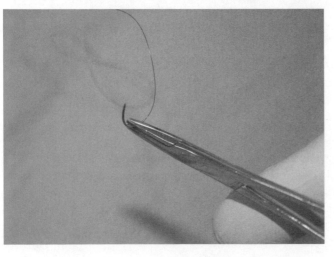

FIGURE 14.2 Proper way to hold the suture needle with the needle holder.

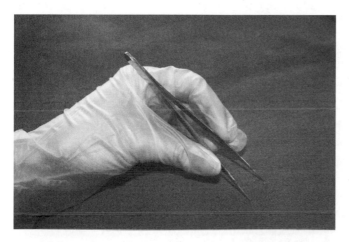

FIGURE 14.3 Holding the forceps

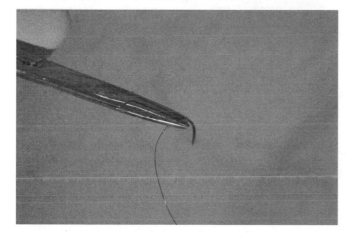

FIGURE 14.4 Inserting the needle at 90°.

- Grab the needle with either the forceps or needle holder, pull through the wound, and reposition the needle holder on the needle as described previously
- Use the forceps to evert the opposite side of the wound
- Push the needle through the inside of the wound adjacent to the first insertion and push through the skin at the same distance from the wound on the opposite side entering the tissue at a 90° angle (Figure 14.5)
- Grab the needle with either the forceps or needle holder
- Pull the material through the tissue leaving a 1- to 2-cm tail
- Place your needle holder parallel to the wound (Figure 14.6A)
- Loop the needle end of the material two times and then grasp the tail with the needle holder and pull across, keeping the twist flat (Figure 14.6B)
- Place the needle holder parallel over the wound and loop one time in the opposite direction
- Grasp the tail and pull across—again, the twist should be flat
  - Approximate the wound edges being careful not to "strangulate" the wound edges (Figure 14.6C)
- Repeat the aforementioned two steps
- Knot(s) should be to the side of the wound and not directly over the wound itself

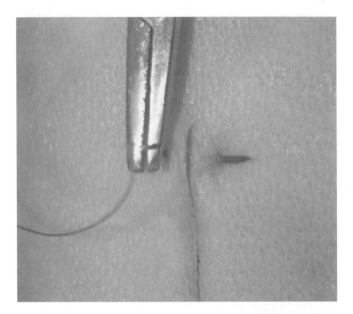

FIGURE 14.5 Needle through the other side.

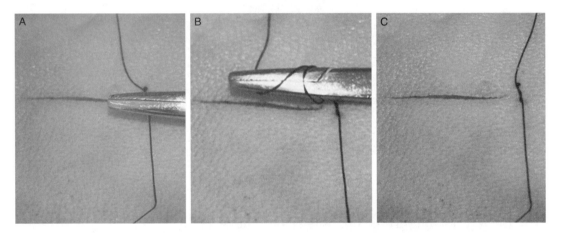

FIGURE 14.6 (A,B,C) Tying a suture knot.

SIMPLE INTERRUPTED SUTURE
- Snip both ends of the material approximately 1 cm above the knot
- Repeat the above steps as many times as needed
- Appropriate spacing (Figure 14.7)
  - Equal space from the entry point to the wound and the wound to the exit
  - Equal space between the sutures
- Where to start
  - Start in the center and work your way out the edges on each side, or start at one end and finish on the opposite side

CONTINUOUS SUTURE (ALSO KNOWN AS A RUNNING SUTURE)
- Snip only the tail end to approximately 1 cm
- Insert the needle beside the first insertion and come out on the other side of the wound

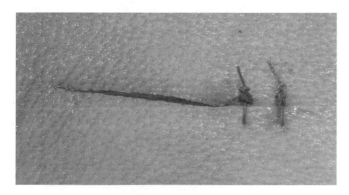

FIGURE 14.7 Appropriate spacing of suture.

- Continue the entire length of the wound
- When you have made your last pass through the wound, do not pull the material all the way through. Leave a loop
- Make a knot as described previously grabbing the loop in place of the free tail. Continuously check the alignment of the unsutured wound edges for potential misalignment, which is known as "dog-ears" (Figure 14.8)
- Continuous sutures take less time but if one area breaks, then they all break. Intermittently locking with a knot can help prevent this from occurring

VERTICAL MATTRESS SUTURE

Best method for everting the wound edges for healing and best used in areas where inversion easily occurs (i.e., palmer surface of hand). This method has two components. The first component is used for wound tension and is deep into the dermis, and the second component is superficial and everts the wound edges. These components allow for a meticulous wound edge approximation.

- Insert the needle slightly farther away than you would for a simple or continuous stitch
- Push through the skin and wound as described previously, keeping the exit the same distance from the wound as the insertion
- Turn the needle around and insert it between the exit and the wound, and come out the other side between the wound edge and the insertion (Figure 14.9)
- Tie a knot as described previously (Figure 14.10)
- Repeat as necessary

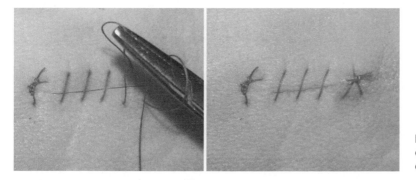

FIGURE 14.8 Making a knot at the end of a continuous suture.

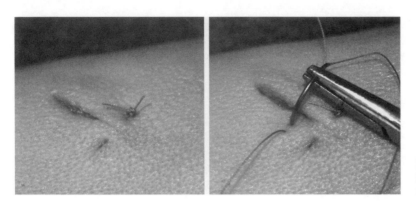

FIGURE 14.9
Performing a vertical mattress.

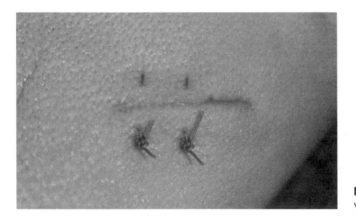

FIGURE 14.10 Completing a vertical mattress suture.

SUBCUTANEOUS SUTURE
- Insert the needle into the dermal layer at one end of the wound and exit toward the center of the wound (Figure 14.11)
- Insert the needle adjacent to the exit and push through adjacent to the first entrance (making a circle)
- Tie a knot as described previously
- Repeat as necessary to close the dermal layer of the wound

SUBCUTICULAR SUTURE (FIGURE 14.12)
- Insert the needle at the base of the subcutaneous tissue and exit just above it
- Insert the needle adjacent to the exit and push through to the base of the subcutaneous layer (adjacent from the first insertion)
- Tie a knot as described previously
- Repeat as necessary to close the deep space

Skin adhesive can be applied or fine percutaneous sutures can be performed to close the percutaneous layer.

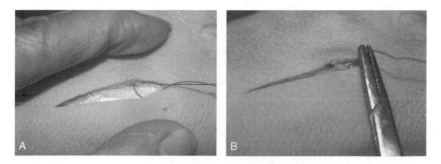

FIGURE 14.11 (A,B) Performing subcutaneous suture.

Staple

The benefits of a staple closure include minimal time required for the procedure, decreased tissue reactivity, and decreased cost compared to suture closure. However, the provider does not have the same control with this method of closure and the staples can interfere with some radiological studies (i.e., CT scan and MRI). Staples should not be used on the face.

- Have an assistant hold the wound edges everted with forceps
- Place the stapler perpendicular to the wound
- Press down as you squeeze the trigger and place the staple
- Repeat as necessary
- Spacing should be equal as with sutures (Figure 14.13)

Skin Adhesive

Skin adhesives are easy to use, painless, and a cost-effective method of closure. However, if you work in an area where water sports and water activities are an everyday or seasonal occurrence, then this method may not be your first choice. Skin adhesives should not get wet, be placed over joints or mobile areas, be placed on wounds with high tension or skin edge distance that have a greater chance of dehiscence than suture or staple closures. Studies have shown that skin adhesives can take

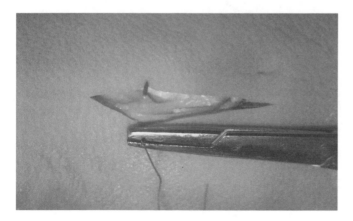

FIGURE 14.12 Performing a subcuticular suture.

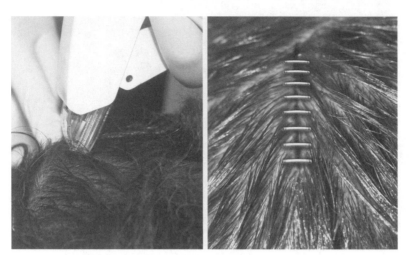

FIGURE 14.13
Performing a staple closure. (Note the equal spacing.)

24 hours to gain full maximum strength and last 5–7 days before tensile strength decreases rapidly secondary to breakdown. They are ideal for superficial and small lacerations. Topical or injectable anesthetics are not required for this method of closure. Studies have shown similar cosmetic outcomes as sutured wounds, making this an advantageous closure technique.

- Irrigate and cleanse the area
- Dry completely
  - Any moisture, including blood, will hinder the skin adhesive from working
- Approximate the wound edges
- Apply the adhesive to the wound. Do NOT place skin adhesive inside the wound as this may cause a foreign body reaction.
- Never place antibiotic ointment or cream over the skin adhesive as it will hasten breakdown
- Skin adhesive cannot be used in high tension wounds unless subcuticular/subcutaneous sutures are placed first
- Allow to dry
- Applying skin tape to the area is optional

Skin Tape

Skin tape is ideal for superficial wounds as well as a re-enforcement of suture, staple, and glue closures. They tend to fall off prematurely and cause the highest rate of wound dehiscence than the other methods when used alone.

- Irrigate and cleanse the wound as described previously
- Dry the area thoroughly
- Dip the cotton-tipped applicator into the benzoin
- Apply to the wound edges
- Allow to dry

- Cut the tape to fit the wounds allowing for approximately 1 cm on each side of the wound
- Approximate the wound edges
- Stick the tape to one side of the wound and gently pull to the other side (this will aid in the approximation)
- Repeat as necessary the entire length of the wound

POSTPROCEDURE CONSIDERATIONS

Bleeding

- Bleeding and "oozing" from a sutured or stapled wound can be common
- Elevate the wound and apply direct pressure
- Light pressure dressings can be applied to the wound

Antibiotic Prophylaxis

- If the wound is older than 8 hours or grossly contaminated, antibiotics should be prescribed unless the wound is on the face or if edges will be excised before closure
- Patients with diabetes, immunosuppression, or on steroids should also be covered with antibiotics

Pain

- Closure, dressings, elevation, and immobilization of joints with wounds will help decrease pain
- Pain medication can be prescribed, if necessary, based on the patient's tolerance and extent of the wound
- Nonsteroidal anti-inflammatory medications should be avoided as they have been linked to delayed healing

EDUCATIONAL POINTS

Wound Care

- Avoid dressing changes for 24 hours to help the healing process and the laying down of granulation tissue
- Instruct the patient to clean with soap and water, and avoid antiseptics (betadyne, alcohol, and hydrogen peroxide) as these can hinder the healing process

Follow-Up

- Wound re-evaluation is recommended in 48 hours
- Follow-up with a specialist is needed for any wounds with tendon, nerve, or deep structure involvement

COMPLICATIONS

- Infection is always a risk even with timely irrigation, closure, and dressing of the wound
- Educating the patient of the possibility of infection and to return if any signs of infection develop is always prudent

AUTHOR'S PEARLS

- *When considering the type of closure, always treat the patient as though he/she is a close family member*
- *When dealing with children and parents remember that this is an anxiety, producing event. Frequent reassurance and a confident attitude go a long way. Even if you don't feel confident, give the performance of your life and it will be better for all involved*
- *When performing a procedure on a child or have a complex wound, try and focus only on the wound. Focusing your concentration takes the pressure off and allows you to treat the wound as any other you have encountered*
- *With jagged, uneven wounds, strategically place sutures. Remember that if you don't like the way it is closing or the tension is not what you expected, there is nothing wrong with removing the suture and replacing it*
- *Open communication with the patient, even when the patient is a child, is very important. Don't ever lie to a patient or parent or try to "candy coat" what you are going to do. They will never trust you again*
- *You can place skin adhesive over sutures to help keep children from pulling knots out*
- *In general, secondary wound infection occurs 24–72 hours after the initial injury. Hence, schedule a 48 hour wound check follow-up*
- *All wounds have a foreign body until proven otherwise with proper exploration*
- *Wound anesthesia should precede wound cleansing*

SPECIAL CONSIDERATIONS/CLOSURES

Lip Laceration Involving the Vermilion Border or Intraoral Cavity

Lip lacerations occur frequently from falls, assaults, animal bites, and motor vehicle crashes. The goal of treatment is a good cosmetic outcome and hemostasis. The lips are composed of three layers: skin, muscle, and oral mucosa. The vermilion border is the area that separates the lip and skin. Unlike facial skin, its stratified squamous epithelium does not contain keratin and has fewer melanocytes. For this reason underlying blood vessels are more apparent; hence the red color. Improper closure can lead to disfigurement. Wounds that are extensive with large pieces of the vermilion border and/or commissure missing (junction where the upper and lower lips join) should always have plastic surgery repair.

PROCEDURE PREPARATION
- Nonsterile gloves
- Absorbable pad
- 4 × 4 gauze
- Skin cleanser
- Topical anesthetic

- Local anesthetic or nerve block (based on location and extent of injury)
- Normal saline for irrigation
- 35–50-mL syringe
- Splash guard or 16–18 gauge angio-catheter
- Surgical scrub
- Suture kit
- Suture material
- Skin tape
- Topical antibiotic

PROCEDURE—LACERATION INVOLVING THE VERMILION BORDER (FIGURE 14.14)
- Place the absorbable pad under the patient's chin
- Cleanse the area
- Apply topical anesthetic
- Perform anesthesia/block
- While the anesthetic takes effect, prepare the other equipment
- Cleanse the area and cover with a fenestrated sterile drape
- Place deep suture as necessary
- Approximate the vermilion border with the first suture using 6–0 nonabsorbable suture material
  - You can also approximate the vermilion border and place a mark with a pen of where you will put the first suture
  - Malalignment of as little as 1 mm can cause disfigurement
- Once the border is aligned, continue your closure using simple interrupted sutures
- Apply topical antibiotic

PROCEDURE—INTRAORAL LACERATION
Any laceration that is gaping, >1.0 cm, or has the potential for food particles to become entrapped should be sutured. The size and depth of the wound will determine how many layers of sutures will be required for closure. If there is a deep space, then internal suture(s) should be performed. Simple interrupted or continuous sutures can be used to close the surface layer with absorbable material.

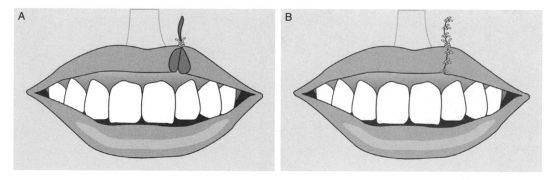

FIGURE 14.14 (A,B) Closure of a lip laceration involving the vermillion border.

Ear Laceration

The ear is unique in that it contains vascular skin tissue covering avascular cartilage tissue. Proper repair of the injury most often results in a good outcome with regard to healing and cosmetic result. Any large avulsions or cartilage involvement should be referred immediately to a plastic surgeon for repair. When small areas of cartilage are involved the area must be debrided and covered with skin for proper healing and outcome which decrease the chance of developing chondritis. The auricular cartilage is avascular and depends on the perichonsrium and surrounding tissue for nutrients. A laceration involving the cartilage is seen in Figure 14.15. Most lacerations of the ear that involve only the skin layers should be closed using the aforementioned methods of closures based on the extent of the laceration. All avascular cartilage must be covered to prevent hematoma formation and promote healing. Local anesthesia must be avoided as it can distort important landmarks. Regional nerve blocks should be used as discussed in Chapter 9. Closing a laceration to the pinna with exposed cartilage will be discussed here.

PROCEDURE PREPARATION
- Nonsterile gloves
- Absorbable pad
- 4 × 4 gauze
- Skin cleanser
- Topical anesthetic
- Local anesthetic or auricular block
- Normal saline for irrigation
- 35–65-mL syringe
- Splash guard or 16–18 gauge angio-catheter

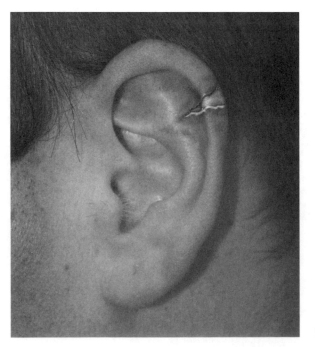

FIGURE 14.15 Wound to pinna.

- Surgical scrub
- Suture kit
- No. 15 scalpel
- Suture material
- Topical antibiotic

PROCEDURE
- Cleanse the area
- Perform anesthetic block (see Chapter 9)
- While the anesthetic takes effect, prepare the other equipment
- Cleanse the area and cover with a fenestrated sterile drape
- With the scalpel, cut a full thickness wedge (triangle) from the antihelix (Figure 14.16A)
- Excise the cartilage
- Because cartilage is so friable and avascular, either do not suture or place sutures through the perichondrium
- Leave 1 mm of overhanging skin to ensure eversion during closure
- With 6–0 nonabsorbable suture material, perform closure (Figure 14.16 B and C)
- Apply a pressure dressing to prevent auricular hematoma
- Close follow-up is required

When closing percutaneous lacerations of the ear not involving the cartilage, close as you would other lacerations but begin posteriorly and end anteriorly. Vertical mattress sutures may be needed when repairing the rim of the ear to ensure eversion.

Nail Bed Laceration

The goal of treatment is to preserve as much tissue as possible, minimize debridement, and prevent further damage/trauma to the nail bed. Educating the patient that the nail may not grow in properly or may never grow is imperative. It can take

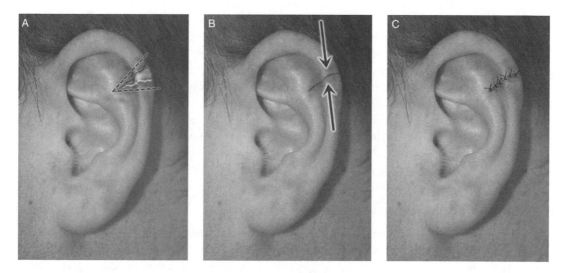

FIGURE 14.16 (A,B,C) Wedge excision and repair of ear laceration.

6 months to 1 year before you know the outcome. The eponychium is the proximal portion of skin at the base of the nail that folds over on itself and supplies the layer of dead skin over the nail plate. If the nail plate is removed during repair, this tissue must not be allowed to come into contact with the nail bed as it will cause scarring and future nail growth disfigurement. Plain radiographs may be necessary to evaluate for underlying tuft or distal phalynx fracture. Children may require conscious sedation to repair the nail bed.

PROCEDURE PREPARATION
- Nonsterile gloves
- Absorbable pad
- 4 × 4 gauze
- Skin cleanser
- Digital block
- Normal saline for irrigation
- 35–65-mL syringe
- Splash guard or 16–18 gauge angio-catheter
- Surgical scrub
- Suture kit
- Suture material
- No. 11 scalpel
- Nonadherent gauze
- Topical antibiotic

PROCEDURE
- Cleanse the area to prepare for a digital block
- Perform a digital block
- While the anesthetic takes effect, prepare the other equipment
- Cleanse the area and cover with a fenestrated sterile drape
- Cut off the tip from a finger of a glove and then cut again
- Place at the base of the finger to aid with hemostasis
- Elevate the nail with either the scalpel or scissors and remove the remainder of the nail
  - Make sure you keep the scissors or scalpel horizontal to the nail bed, being careful not to cause further damage/trauma to the nail bed
- Once the nail is lifted, remove with a hemostat/needle holder
- Irrigate the nail bed with normal saline and debride any devitalized tissue
- Place the sutures using 6-0 absorbable suture material
- Once you have finished with the sutures, reapply the nail by placing a 4-0 nonabsorbable suture through the nail on each side of the base of the nail and securing it to the surrounding skin (Figure 14.17)
- Apply a dry sterile dressing and splint as necessary

Tendon Lacerations

Flexor tendon lacerations usually involve the synovial membrane and should always be handled by a hand specialist immediately. Repair of the tendon should not be attempted due to the risk of tenosynovitis. Debridement with copious irrigation

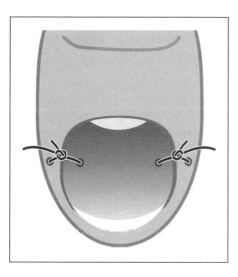

FIGURE 14.17 Securing the nail after repair of a nail bed laceration.

should be performed. Extensor tendons do not possess the synovial membrane and can be either repaired or closed over after debridement and copious irrigation and referred for follow-up with a hand specialist. Flexor tendons possess a synovial membrane and repair should be done by a specialist.

RESOURCES

Brown, D. J., Jaffe, J. E., & Henson, J. K. (2007). *Emergency medical clinics of North America, 25,* 83–99.

Bruns, T. B., & Worthington, J. M. (2000). Using tissue adhesive for wound repair: A practical guide to dermabond. *American Family Physician, 61*(5), 1383–1388. Retrieved from http://www.aafp.org/afp/20000301/1383.html

DeSouza, B. A., Shibu, M., Moir, G., Carver, N., Dunn, R., Watson, S., et al. (2002). Suturing v conservative management of hand lacerations. *British Medical Journal, 325,* 1113–1117.

Fansler, J. L., & Schreibner, D. (2010, January 14). Complex laceration, lip. Retrieved from http://emedicine.medscape.com/article/83256-overview & http://emedicine.medscape.com/article/83256-treatment

Hollander, J. E. (2003). Wound closure options. In A. J. Singer & J. E. Hollander (Eds.), *Lacerations and acute wounds: An evidence-based guide* (pp. 56–63). Philadelphia: F. A. Davis Company.

Hollander, J. E. (2003). Selecting sutures and needles for wound closure. In A. J. Singer & J. E. Hollander (Eds.), *Lacerations and acute wounds: An evidence-based guide* (pp. 98–107). Philadelphia: F. A. Davis Company.

Hollander, J. E., & Singer, A. J. (1999). Laceration management. *Annals of Emergency Medicine, 34,* 356–367.

Jolly, J. (2009). Surgical staples for scalp laceration repair: A quick and easy solution. *Advance for Nurse Practitioners, 17*(7), 37–38.

Kumar, K. (2009, October 13). Complex laceration, ear. Retrieved from http://emedicine.medscape.com/article/83294-overview & http://emedicine.medscape.com/article/83294-treatment

Lammers, R. L. (2010). Principles of wound management. In J. R. Roberts & J. R. Hedges, (Eds.), *Clinical procedures in emergency medicine* (5th ed.). Philadelphia: Saunders Elsevier.

Quinn, J., Cummings, S., Callaham, M., & Sellers, K. (2002). Suturing versus conservative management of lacerations of the hand: Randomized controlled trial. *British Medical Journal, 325,* 299. Retrieved from http://bmj.com/cgi/content/full/325/7359/299?view=l ong&pmid=12169503

Singer, A. J. (2003). Adhesive tapes. In A. J. Singer & J. E. Hollander (Eds.), *Lacerations and acute wounds: An evidence-based guide* (pp. 64–72). Philadelphia: F. A. Davis Company.

Singer, A. J. (2003). Surgical staples. In A. J. Singer & J. E. Hollander (Eds.),. *Lacerations and acute wounds: An evidence-based guide* (pp. 73–82). Philadelphia: F. A. Davis Company.

Singer, A. J., & Hollander, J. E. (2003). Wound preparation. In A. J. Singer, & J. E. Hollander (Eds.), *Lacerations and acute wounds: An evidence-based guide* (pp. 13–22). Philadelphia: F. A. Davis Company.

Singer, A. J., & Quinn, J. V. (2003). Tissue adhesive. In A. J. Singer & J. E. Hollander (Eds.), *Lacerations and acute wounds: An evidence-based guide* (pp. 83–97). Philadelphia: F. A. Davis Company.

Sodovsky, R. (2000). Management of lacerations to avoid infection and scarring. Retrieved from www.aafp.org/afp/20000301/tips/33.html

Sutijono, D., & Silverberg, M. A. (2009, May 7). Nailbed injuries. Retrieved from http://emedicine.medscape.com/article/827104-overview&http://emedicine.medscape.comarticle/827104-treatment

Thomsen, T. W., Barclay, D. A., & Setnik, G. S. (2006). Basic laceration repair. *New England Journal of Medicine, 355*(17), e18.

Trott, A. T. (2005). Wound cleansing and irrigation. In *Wounds and lacerations: Emergency care and closure* (3rd ed., pp. 83–92). Philadelphia: Mosby Elsevier.

Trott, A. T. (2005). Instruments and suture material. In *Wounds and lacerations: Emergency care and closure* (3rd ed., pp. 93–106). Philadelphia: Mosby Elsevier.

Trott, A. T. (2005). Basic laceration repair: Principles and techniques. In *Wounds and lacerations: Emergency care and closure* (3rd ed., pp. 119–134). Philadelphia: Mosby Elsevier.

Trott, A. T. (2005). Special anatomical sites. In *Wounds and lacerations: Emergency care and closure* (3rd ed., pp. 153–176). Philadelphia: Mosby Elsevier.

Wang, Q. C., & Johnson, B. A. (2001). Fingertip injuries. *American Family Physicians, 63*(10), 1961–1966.

Managing Minor Burns

Theresa M. Campo

BACKGROUND

Burns can cause devastation and even death. The purpose of this chapter is to outline the type, degree, and treatment of minor burns, including sunburn. Acute management of any burn is to immediately stop the burn from causing further damage and to initiate prompt treatment, and arrange referral as necessary. Always assess for the potential severe associated injury. For instance, a patient who presents from a fire should be evaluated for smoke inhalation (burned or singed nasal hairs, hoarse voice, cough, etc.). Follow-up is imperative with burns to reduce the risk of infection, scarring, and loss of function.

Traditionally, burns were classified as first-, second-, and third-degree burns. Today the burns are classified by the depth and extent of the burn. The current classifications are epidermal, partial thickness (superficial or deep), and full thickness. The current classifications correspond with the traditional.

Epidermal burns, or first degree burns, are painful, red, and moist. Blistering does not occur and the damage is mostly to the epidermal layer of skin. Healing usually occurs in 5 to 7 days with no scarring. The most common epidermal burn is sunburn. Partial thickness burns can be either superficial or deep. Superficial partial thickness burns involve the epidermal layer and several dermal layers of the skin. They are painful and heal, usually with minimal scarring, in 2 to 3 weeks. Deep partial thickness burns involve the epidermal and dermal layers and may involve some of the dermal appendages. They are not as painful as epidermal or superficial partial thickness burns because of the loss of sensory nerves. Sensation to pinpricks is intact. Healing can be more than 3 weeks with increased scarring. Full thickness burns involve the entire epidermal and dermal layers of skin. They are dry, leathery, and insensitive. Patients present with little or no pain. The color of the burn can be white, brown, or black. These burns cause significant scarring, loss of function, and usually require skin grafting. Deep partial thickness and full thickness burns may be difficult to distinguish during the initial evaluation.

The depth and body surface area (BSA) have a direct impact on healing and mortality of burns. The rating of burns can be done using the "rule of nines," which designates a percentage to certain anatomical locations. The head and each arm account for 9% each; the genitals equal 1%; and the anterior, posterior trunk, and each leg account for 18% each. The percentages for children using the rule of nines are more specific (Figure 15.1).

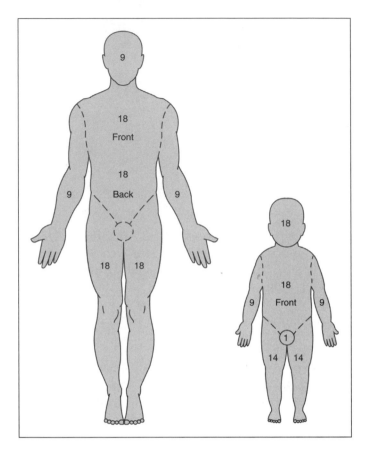

FIGURE 15.1 Rule of nines.

A more practical way to ascertain the percentage of BSA burned is to take the palm of the patient's hand, which equals 1%. This is a practical and accurate way to estimate the BSA without using calculations and diagrams (Figure 15.2).

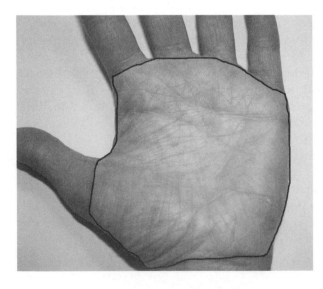

FIGURE 15.2 Palm of hand = 1% BSA.

PATIENT PRESENTATION

Epidermal

- Painful
- Red
- No blisters

Superficial Partial Thickness

- Very painful
- Red
- Blanches with pressure
- Moist
- Weeping
- Blister may or may not be present (usually intact if present)

Deep Partial Thickness

- Pain
- Perception of pressure
- Waxy appearance

Full Thickness

- Not painful
- Perception of deep pressure
- Waxy white or gray color

TREATMENT

Treatment is based on depth, cause, and body surface affected. The goal of treatment is to quickly stop the burn, identify the extent of the burn, and administer pain medication immediately. Many patients will present with "home remedies" for treating burns. These can include butter, ketchup, petroleum jelly, and submersion in a bucket of ice. Although you want to cool the burn, ice cubes can attach to and tear off blistered skin. Always be careful with removal of anything that is touching the skin including clothing, towels, and gauze. Cooling a burn can be effective for up to 3 hours after the initial injury. Applying a moist cool towel can minimize tissue damage.

Burns that require hospitalization and/or referral to a burn center are as follows:

Partial and Full Thickness Burns

- Partial thickness
  - Burns covering 15% BSA—adults
  - 10% BSA—children
- Full thickness
  - Burns of greater than 3% BSA
  - Partial or full thickness burns of the face, genitals, hands, or feet

- Any partial or full thickness burn to the face, genitals, hands, and feet (especially if circumferential)
- Electrical burns
- Smoke inhalation
- Suspected child abuse
- Age either greater than 65 years or younger than 2 years
- Patients who are immunocompromised or have diabetes, or those patients taking chemotherapeutics or immunosuppressive medications should also be considered for hospitalization or referral to a burn center

Any burns involving the face, hands, feet, and genitalia should be referred to a burn center. Burns that are circumferential on the hands, feet, or penis should be transferred to a burn center immediately.

SPECIAL CONSIDERATIONS

- Diabetes
- Immunosuppression
- Chemotherapeutics
- Anticoagulation
- History of electrolyte imbalance

PROCEDURE PREPARATION

- Sterile water or normal saline for irrigating
- Silver sulfadiazine (Silvadene)
  - Do not use on the face
- Topical antibiotic ointment (polymixin, bacitracin)
  - Use on face
- Use mupirocin (Bactroban) if sulfa allergic. Both silver sulfadiazine and other topical antibiotics contain sulfa
- Nonadherent gauze
- 2 × 2 or 4 × 4 gauze (depending on area)
- Loose roll gauze (Kerlix)
- Tape

PROCEDURE

- Medicate for pain
  - Partial and full thickness burns usually require narcotic pain medication either oral or parenteral
- Cleanse the area to remove any products applied by the patient or other persons prior to arrival
- Dry completely
- Debride the area of any loose tissue and open blisters
- Apply silver sulfadiazine
- Cover with nonadherent gauze
- Place 2 × 2 or 4 × 4 gauze over the nonadherent gauze

- Loosely wrap the rolled gauze over the area
- Do not apply dressings tightly. This can cause further damage

POSTPROCEDURE CONSIDERATIONS

- Pain medication should be prescribed
- Close follow-up with the burn center, plastic surgeon, or primary care provider

EDUCATIONAL POINTS

- Dressing changes should be done at least once daily and optimally twice daily with silver sulfadiazine
- Elevation will assist with reducing swelling

COMPLICATIONS

- Infection
- Contracture
- Scarring

AUTHOR'S PEARLS

- *Educate the patient to completely cleanse the silver sulfadiazine before the next application. The medication has the potential to pigment the skin. This is why it isn't recommended for use on the face*
- *Circumferential burns of the hands, feet, or body in children should be suspected for child abuse*

RESOURCES

Bethel, C. A., & Mazzeo, A. S. Burn care procedures. (2009). In J. R. Roberts & J. R. Hedges (Eds.), *Clinical procedures in emergency medicine* (5th ed.). (pp. 692–714) Philadelphia: Saunders Elsevier.

Caron, A., & McStay, C. M. (2009, May 18). Sunburn. Retrieved from http://emedicine.medscape.com/article/773203-overview & http://emedicine.medscape.com/article/773203-treatment

Goodis, J., & Schraga, E. D. (2009, June 28). Burns, thermal. Retrieved from http://emedicine.medscape.com/article/769193-overview & http://emedicine.medscape.com/article/769193-treatment

Lafferty, K. A. (2009, December 9). Smoke inhalation. Retrieved from http://emedicine.medscape.com/article/771194-overview

Morgan, E. D., Bledsoe, S. C., & Barker, J. (2000). Ambulatory management of burns. *American Family Physician,* Retrieved from http://www.aafp.org/afp/20001101/2015.html

Soroff, H. S., & Brebbia, J. S. (2003). Burns. In A. J. Singer & J. E. Hollander (Eds). *Lacerations and acute wounds: An evidence-based guide* (pp. 173–187). Philadelphia: F. A. Davis Company.

Trott, A. T. (2005). Minor burns. In *Wounds and lacerations: Emergency care and closure* (3rd ed., pp. 253–262). Philadelphia: Mosby Elsevier.

Procedure for Managing Ingrown Toe Nails

THERESA M. CAMPO

BACKGROUND

Toe nails mainly consist of the proximal nail fold, cuticle, nail plate, hyponychium, and nail bed. The proximal nail fold covers one-fifth of the base of the nail and protects the nail matrix, which lies below. The cuticle or eponychium is formed from the proximal nail fold and attaches to the nail plate acting as a protector against microorganisms. The nail plate extends to the hyponychium (thick skin just below the distal nail plate). The nail bed facilitates the smooth movement of the nail plate distally, but does not participate in the actual nail development. It supports the nail and contains blood vessels and nerves. The nail matrix (root) is solely responsible for the formation and growth of the nail plate (Figures 16.1 and 16.2). Nails grow 1 mm in a month.

Normal nail growth is distal from the proximal nail fold and should be smooth. However, lateral growth of the nail plate into the soft tissue causes an inflammatory response. Ingrown toe nails are most commonly the result of improperly fitting shoes and improper nail cutting. It can also be the result of increased age, pregnancy, repetitive trauma, hyperhidrosis, poor hygiene, improper nail grooming, or underlying disorders (i.e., diabetes, immunosuppression, obesity, thyroid disease, cardiac disease, and renal disorders). The shape of nail growth can place a person at risk to develop infected ingrown nails. The most common site is the great toe.

The severity of the ingrown nail and reaction to this form of growth can range from mild to severe. A mild presentation may consist of swelling, edema, and hyperkeratosis, whereas a moderate presentation consists of increased edema, drainage, pain, infection, and ulceration of the nail fold. Severe cases progress to increased production of granulation tissue with layering over the nail plate. This may be accompanied by infection and severe pain.

A study by De Berker et al. (2008) described a retronychia, which is the proximal ingrowing of the nail plate and is associated with multiple generations of nail plates. The most common cause was distal nail trauma from footwear pushing the nail back and upward. This pushes the proximal nail above the new growth. As the new nail grows, it displaces the previous nail growth upward rather than advancing it forward. The nail becomes thickened and discolored from the layering of nails. Granulation is common with retronychia.

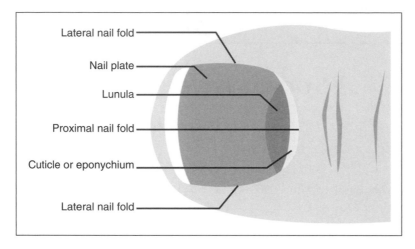

FIGURE 16.1 Anatomy of a toe nail.

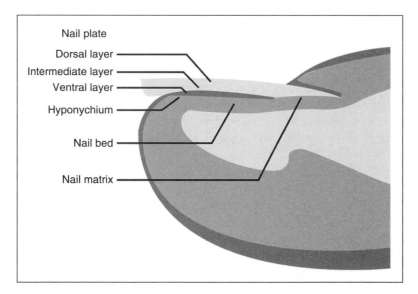
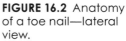

FIGURE 16.2 Anatomy of a toe nail—lateral view.

PATIENT PRESENTATION

- Throbbing pain
- Edema
- Erythema
- Purulent drainage
- Granulation tissue
- Foul smell

TREATMENT

Treatment is based on the severity of the ingrown toe nail. The goal of treatment is to decrease pain and inflammation as well as promote normal nail growth. Mild cases are treated with cold soaks, steroids, 20% to 40% topical urea cream (Keralac, Carmol), cotton wisps under the lateral nail plate, and gutter splinting. Cases not responsive to conservative therapy may require removal of the nail spicule with or without a portion of the nail. Lateral matrixectomy may also be necessary. Matrixectomy is the removal of the nail matrix. This is done by manually removing the nail matrix with or without either silver nitrate, electrocautery, or a chemical solution such as phenol or 10% sodium hydroxide solution.

Infected ingrown toe nails are most commonly caused by *Staphylococcus aureus*, streptococcus, and gram-negative bacteria (i.e., pseudomonas). If antibiotic treatment is necessary, then coverage for these organisms should be considered.

CONTRAINDICATIONS AND RELATIVE CONTRAINDICATIONS

- Allergy to local anesthetics
- Bleeding dyscrasia
- Diabetic patients with neuropathic disease should not have matrixectomy performed

SPECIAL CONSIDERATIONS

- Diabetics
- Immunocompromised

PROCEDURE PREPARATION

Minor Ingrown Toenail

- Gloves (nonsterile)
- Skin tape strips (Steri-strips)
- Small gauze angiocatheter

Moderate to Severe Ingrown Toenail

- Absorbent pads
- Skin cleanser
- 3-ml syringe with small-gauge needle (25–30 gauge) filled with lidocaine or bupivacaine
- Sterile gauze
- Bone curette
  - Tissue nipper if unavailable
- English anvil nail splitter
  - Small pointed scissors
- Forceps or hemostat
- Penrose drain
- Silver nitrate sticks
  - Aqueous phenol solution (1%) or sodium hydroxide solution (10%) if available
- Cotton-tipped applicator
  - Some of the cotton can be removed to fit the small area of the excised wound
- Topical antibiotic ointment
  - Topical antibiotic cream (i.e., silver sulfadiazine [Silvadene]) should be used if chemical solution or silver nitrate used

- Nonadherent gauze dressing
- Roll gauze

PROCEDURE

Minor Ingrown Toenail

MINIMAL INFLAMMATION AND NO GRANULATION TISSUE
- Warm soaks
- Place a skin tape strip (Steri-strip) under the affected section of the nail and secure to the toe (Figure 16.3)
  - You can also place a small piece of tubing (small-gauge angiocath cut to fit the area) around the lateral nail on the nail spicule and tape into place with a skin tape strip

Moderate Ingrown Toenail

INFLAMMATION ACCOMPANIED BY GRANULATION TISSUE
Oblique section of nail removal for nails with inflammation and little to no granulation tissue.

- Cleanse the skin using a circular motion to free debris and bacteria
- Place an absorbent protective pad under the treatment area
- Digital block (see Chapter 5)
- Clean the area of granulation tissue with a bone curette to expose the offending nail border
- Remove an oblique section from the distal corner of the nail using the English anvil nail splitters (Figure 16.4)
  - Small pointed scissors can be used with upward pressure and a controlled push method to minimize nail bed trauma
  - One-third to one-half distal to proximal nail fold

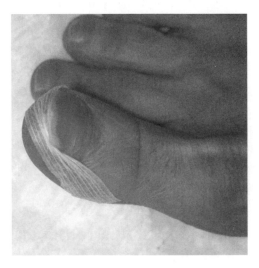

FIGURE 16.3 Skin closure (Steri-strip) under nail.

- Grab the cut portion of nail with forceps or hemostats and remove
- Gently debride the area with either the forceps or hemostat
- Silver nitrate can be applied if there is any residual bleeding
- Dress the wound with antibiotic ointment and nonadherent gauze
  - Topical antibiotic cream (i.e., silver sulfadiazine [Silvadene]) should be used if chemical solution or silver nitrate used

Moderate to Severe Ingrown Toenail

INFLAMMATION WITH GRANULATION TISSUE

Nail removal can be either partial or complete. Complete nail removal is rarely needed unless both lateral nail folds are involved. This should be referred to a podiatric specialist.

- Cleanse the skin using a circular motion to free debris and bacteria
- Place an absorbent protective pad under the treatment area
- Digital block (see Chapter 5)
- Apply Penrose drain to the base of the toe
- Mark the lateral quarter to one-third of the nail on the affected side (Figure 16.5)
- Lift the nail with either forceps or hemostat
- Using the English anvil nail splitter, cut the nail distal to proximal just past the proximal cuticle
  - The cut should not be farther than two-thirds of the nail distal to proximal to prevent nail bed damage
- With small sharp scissors cut the final one-third of the nail to just beneath the cuticle (a few millimeters)
- Grab the cut nail with forceps or hemostat
- Pull the loose piece while rotating away from the lateral edge and toward the intact nail removing it from its attachment
- Inspect the area for any remaining pieces of nail
- Debride the area of any loose nail fragments or hyperkeratotic tissue with the forceps

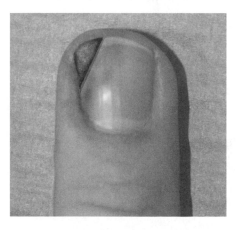

FIGURE 16.4 Oblique section removal.

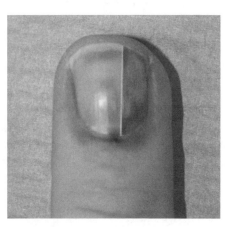

FIGURE 16.5 Partial nail removal.

Matrixectomy

Debridement of the granulation tissue is usually sufficient and does not require matrixectomy. Consultation with podiatry should be considered if this procedure is necessary and performed.

Note: Silver nitrate, electrocautery, or chemical solutions (phenol, 10% sodium hydroxide solution) can be used for this procedure.

SILVER NITRATE
- Apply silver nitrate to the granulation tissue for 2 to 3 minutes

ELECTROCAUTERY
- Apply to granulation tissue

PHENOL (SHOULD NOT BE USED IF INFECTION IS PRESENT)
- Soak a cotton-tipped applicator with phenol
- Apply to area of nail matrix for 30 seconds
  - Use a rolling motion to avoid damage to nail edge or viable surrounding tissue
- Repeat two times
- Irrigate the area to remove phenol
- It is important to keep the area clean and dry during the application of a chemical solution/agent

10% SODIUM HYDROXIDE SOLUTION (SHOULD NOT BE USED IF INFECTION IS PRESENT)
- Soak a cotton-tipped applicator with 10% sodium hydroxide solution
- Apply to the area of nail matrix for 30 seconds
  - Use a rolling motion to avoid damage to nail edge
- Repeat two times
- Irrigate the area to remove the solution
- Do not forget to remove the Penrose drain (tourniquet)
- Apply silver sulfadiazine (Silvadene) and a nonadherent dressing with rolled gauze (Kling)
- It is important to keep the area clean and dry during the application of a chemical solution/agent

POSTPROCEDURE CONSIDERATIONS

Pain

- Ingrown nails may be exquisitely tender and digital block should be performed slowly and with a small-gauge needle (i.e., 25 to 30 gauge)
- Scissors can be used in place of the English anvil nail splitter
- If phenol or other ablating solutions are available, they can be used in place of the silver nitrate. These substances will prevent further nail growth

EDUCATIONAL POINTS

Minor Ingrown Toe Nails

- Warm water soaks with epsom salt 2 to 3 times daily

- Wound evaluation 48 to 72 hours after procedure
  - Diabetic or immunocompromised patients or patients with peripheral vascular disease should be followed more closely with strong consideration of prophylactic antibiotic use
- Patients with ingrown nails caused by deformity should be referred to a podiatrist for definitive nail removal

Moderate Ingrown Toe Nails

- Warm water soaks 2 to 3 times daily
- Dry dressing
- Healing occurs within 2 to 4 weeks

COMPLICATIONS

- Complications are minimal but regrowth of the nail, infection or extending infection (abscess), osteomyelitis and delayed healing, and recurrence are all possibilities

---

AUTHOR'S PEARLS

- *Cutting the finger of a latex/rubber glove can be used as a tourniquet in place of a Penrose drain*
- *If English anvil nail splitters are not available, iris scissors can be used. However, be sure not to cut or damage the nail bed*
- *Use the "push–pull" method gentle controlled use of the scissor while inserting under the nail plate*

RESOURCES

Benzoni, T. E. (2010, March 15). Toenails, ingrown. Retrieved from http://emedicine.medscape.com/article/828072-overview & http://emedicine.medscape.com/article/828072-treatment

Chavez, M. C., & Maker, V. K. (2007). Office surgery. In R. E. Rakel (Ed.), *Textbook of family medicine* (7th ed.). Philadelphia: Saunders Elsevier. Retrieved from http://www.mdconsult.com/das/book/body/187327964-5/963237221/1481/390.html#4-u1.0-B978-1-4160-2467-5..50036-1–cesec68_1821

De Berker, D. A., Richert, B., Duhard, E., Piraccini, B. M., Andre, J., & Baran, R. (2008). Retronychia: Proximal ingrowing of the nail plate. *Journal of the American Academy of Dermatology, 58*, 978–983.

Habif, T. P. (2009). Nail diseases. In *Clinical dermatology: A color guide to diagnosis and treatment* (5th ed.). Retrieved from http://www.mdconsult.com/book/player/book.do?method=display&type=bookPage&decorator=header&eid=4-u1.0-B978-0-7234-3541-9..00034-1–s0315&displayedEid=4-u1.0-B978-0-7234-3541-9..00034-1–s0350&uniq=187327964&isbn=978-0-7234-3541-9&sid=963240480

Heidelbaugh, J. L., & Lee, H. (2009). Management of the ingrown toenail. *American Family Physician, 79*(4), 303–308, 311–312.

McGee, D. L. (2009). Podiatric procedures. In J. R. Roberts & J. R. Hedges, (Eds.), *Clinical procedures in emergency medicine* (5th ed., pp. 939–943). Philadelphia: Saunders Elsevier.

Mostaghimi, L. (2010). Diseases of the skin: Diseases of the nails. In E. T. Bope, R. E. Rakel, & R. D. Kellerman (Eds.), *Conn's current therapy 2010* (1st ed.). Retrieved from http://www.mdconsult.com/book/player/book.do?method=display&type=bookPage&decorator=header&eid=4-u1.0-B978-1-4160-6642-2..00013-2–s0845&uniq=187327964&isbn=978-1-4160-6642-2&sid=963240480

Richardson, E. G. (2008). Disorders of nails and skin. In S. T. Canale & J. H. Beaty (Eds.), *Campbell's operative orthopaedics* (11th ed.). Retrieved from http://www.mdconsult.com/das/book/body/187327964-6/963237528/1584/638.html#4-u1.0-B978-0-323-03329-9..50087-8–cesec1_4367

Schraga, E. D. (2009, November 10). Ingrown toenail removal. Retrieved from http://emedicine.medscape.com/article/149627-overview&http://emedicine.medscape.com/article/149627-treatment.

Xuber, T. J. (2002). Ingrown toenail removal. *American Family Physician, 65*(12), 2547–2550.

Procedures for Treating Subungual Hematoma

Theresa M. Campo

BACKGROUND

A subungual hematoma is a collection of blood between the nail plate and nail bed. It is often caused by a crushing injury or blunt trauma to the distal aspect of a digit, causing accumulation of blood under the nail plate, in turn causing pressure and pain. The degree of the hematoma may be minimal or severe with or without coin ciding distal phalanx or tuft fractures.

Pain is the most common complaint and can be relieved quickly by performing trephination to the nail.

PATIENT PRESENTATION

- Throbbing, painful finger
- Dark red to black coloration to nail

TREATMENT

The treatment of a subungual hematoma is dependent upon the amount of the nail that is affected. If the hematoma is small (<25%) and painless, then treatment is usually not required. However, if the hematoma covers more than 25% of the nail bed and pain is present, then decompression (trephination) should be performed. If the hematoma covers more than 50% of the nail, then removal of the nail should be considered and any laceration to the nail bed should be repaired. Approximately 50% of subungual hematomas covering 50% or more of the nail have associated nail bed laceration injuries. The incidence increases significantly when associated with a distal tuft fracture. Repair of nail bed lacerations is discussed in Chapter 14.

CONTRAINDICATIONS AND RELATIVE CONTRAINDICATIONS

There are no contraindications or relative contraindications for this procedure.

SPECIAL CONSIDERATIONS

- Associated nail bed laceration
- Associated distal phalanx and/or tuft fractures

PROCEDURE PREPARATION

Heat Method

- Cautery stick (may use a heated paper clip)
- Gauze

Drilling Method

- 18-gauge needle
- Gauze

PROCEDURE

- Cleanse the skin using a circular motion to remove debris and bacteria
- Place an absorbent protective pad under the treatment area
- Drape the patient to maintain a clean area as well as protect the patient's privacy
- Strict sterile technique is not required for this procedure. However, because of the era of resistance, sterile technique should be used whenever possible

Heat Method

- Hold the cautery stick perpendicular to the nail plate
- Once it is heated and ready, press the tip through the nail plate (Figure 17.1)
- Once it penetrates the nailplate and hematoma, the blood will drain and cool the tip preventing damage to the nailbed
- Apply pressure to the nail and finger to drain the hematoma

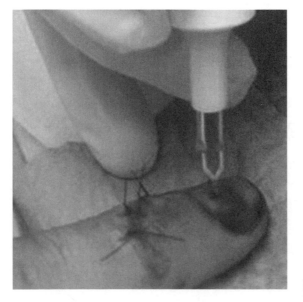

FIGURE 17.1 Trephination—heat method.

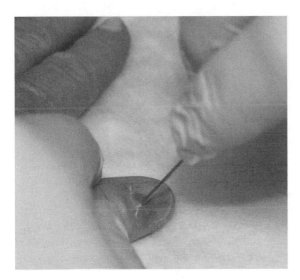

FIGURE 17.2 Trephination—drill method.

Drilling Method

- Take the 18-gauge needle and press through the nail plate with gentle pressure while rotating the needle in a circular motion (Figure 17.2)
  - Be careful not to penetrate the nailbed as this is a common complication with this method

POSTPROCEDURE CONSIDERATIONS

Pain

- Digital block can be performed if patient is intolerant of procedure
- Instruct the patient to keep the finger elevated, above the level of the heart, to prevent throbbing and pain

EDUCATIONAL POINTS

- Elevation
- Clean with soap and water
- Apply topical antibiotic
- Systemic antibiotic therapy is not warranted but should be considered with an open tuft or phalanx fracture
- Consideration should be given to children with a significant or recurring hematoma, and child abuse should be ruled out
- A device approved by the Food and Drug Administration called the Path Former can decrease the amount of trauma during trephination with more concise control

COMPLICATIONS

- Infection

AUTHOR'S PEARLS

■ *Tube gauze may be used to give light pressure and encourage drainage*
■ *The heat method is preferred because of the potential nail bed trauma with the drill method*

RESOURCES

Huang, Y. H., & Ohara, K. (2005). Medical pearl: Subungual hematoma: A simple and quick method for diagnosis. *Journal of the American Academy of Dermatology, 54,* 877–878.

Lammers, R. L. (2010). Methods of wound care. In J. R. Roberts & J. R. Hedges (Eds.), *Clinical procedures in emergency medicine* (5th ed., pp. 626). Philadelphia: Saunders Elsevier.

Procedures for Managing Paronychia

Theresa M. Campo

BACKGROUND

Paronychia is a superficial infection of the nail fold. It is most commonly caused by frequent nail biting or chewing of the periungual tissue and by an aggressive manicure. Paronychia is one of the most common infections of the hand.

Paronychia can be either acute or chronic. Acute paronychia usually affects one digit and is characterized by acute onset of pulsating pain, swelling, and erythema of the periungual space, usually unilateral. Chronic paronychia is caused by frequent and increased water exposure, humidity, detergents, and irritants, which cause irritation and maceration of the proximal nail fold. This leads to inflammation, swelling of the nail fold, and cessation of cuticle production. The most common organisms found in chronic paronychia are *Candida albicans* and *Pseudomonas aeruginosa*. Acute paronychia will be discussed in detail in this chapter.

Most Common Pathogens Causing Acute Paronychia

- *Streptococcus pyogenes*
- *Staphylococcus aureus*
- *Eikenella corrodens*
- Anaerobic organisms
  - *Provotella* spp.
  - *Fusobacterium nucleatum*
  - Gram-positive cocci
  - *Peptostreptococcus* spp.

Note: Practitioners should always consider mixed oropharyngeal flora as the causative organism.

Paronychia can be confused with a herpetic whitlow. This infection is most often seen in health care workers and immunocompromised patients. The most common presentation is localized swelling with clear vesicles. Lymphangitis, lymphadenopathy, and a dusky appearance to the nail may also be present. Viral culture should be obtained if possible and sent for Tzanck smear and serum antibody titers. Opening of the vesicles is not recommended. This infection is self-limiting and should resolve within 3 to 4 weeks.

PATIENT PRESENTATION

■ Warm, erythematous, edematous, and painful unilateral or bilateral lateral nail fold
■ Frank abscess and occasional extension to the eponychia can occur
■ Lymphangitis and lymphadenopathy are usually not seen

TREATMENT

Early paronychia is characterized by redness and mild swelling. Treatment is localized and noninvasive. Warm soaks, elevation, and antibiotic therapy with dicloxacillin or cephalexin are recommended. More extensive infection with fluctuance requires drainage of the pustulent material. This procedure will be covered in this chapter.

SPECIAL CONSIDERATIONS

■ Diabetics
■ Immunocompromised

PROCEDURE PREPARATION

■ Absorbent pad
■ Skin cleanser
■ No. 11 or No. 15 scalpel blade with handle
■ Scissors
■ Culture swab
■ Normal saline solution
■ Large syringe (20-, 30-, or 35-mL)
■ Gauze pads
■ Kling or gauze for wrapping
■ Tape

PROCEDURE

■ Place an absorbent protective pad under the treatment area
■ Cleanse the skin using a circular motion to free debris and bacteria
■ Drape the patient to maintain a clean area
■ Strict sterile technique is not required for this procedure. However, because of the era of resistance, sterile technique should be used whenever possible

   Note: Ethyl chloride or a digital block can be used based on the patient's pain tolerance and extent of the paronychia

Localized Pus Collection

■ Position an 18-gauge needle bevel up and parallel to the nail surface
■ Insert the needle into the lateral nailfold at the point of maximum fluctuance (Figure 18.1)
■ Lift the skin of the nail fold, which will release the pus

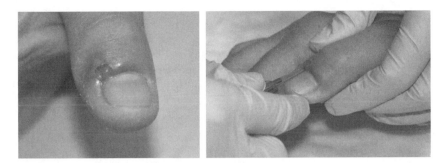

FIGURE 18.1 Releasing localized pus collection of a paronychia.

- Use a gentle side-to-side motion and "fan out" the area allowing full expression of the contents
- Obtain culture
- Soak or irrigate with normal saline
  - Irrigate with syringe and splash shield
- Insert packing if possible
- Apply sterile dressing

Complex

- Perform digital block technique (see Chapter 7)
- Holding the scalpel parallel to the nail surface and gently advance the scalpel under the eponychium making sure not to invade the nailbed (Figure 18.2)
- Express the contents
- Irrigate with normal saline
- Insert packing
- Apply sterile dressing

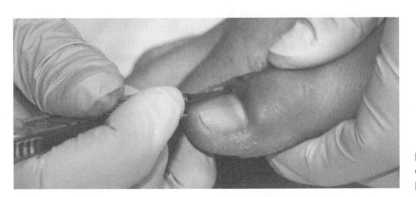

FIGURE 18.2 Incision and drainage of paronychia.

POSTPROCEDURE CONSIDERATIONS

Pain

- Digital block can be performed if patient is intolerant of the procedure
- Instruct the patient to keep the finger elevated, above the level of the heart, to prevent throbbing and pain

Drainage

- If the paronychia is small, you may only get a very small amount of drainage
- Consider herpetic whitlow if pus drainage is less than expected based on the amount of swelling and presentation

Ingrown Nail

- If an ingrown nail is present or the pus collection is under the nail, lifting the nail may be necessary or a semilunar incision proximal to the nail fold may be required

Mobile Nail

- If the nail is mobile, removal may be necessary

EDUCATIONAL POINTS

- Elevation
- Clean with soap and water
- Apply topical antibiotic
- Incision and drainage is the ideal treatment of paronychia
- Systemic antibiotic therapy is not always warranted
- Instruct patients not to bite or chew nails, to be careful with aggressive manicures, and not to suck on fingers

COMPLICATIONS

- Progression of infection to surrounding tissue causing cellulitis, lymphangitis, and/ or fever should be treated with antibiotic therapy
- Recurrence of the abscess necessitates consideration of risk factors or abnormalities including foreign body, cancer, staph. colonization, and immunologic disorders

Author's Pearl

- *Ethyl chloride can be used topically to decrease the pain experienced with incision or puncture of the pustule*

RESOURCES

Browning, J., & Levy, M., & Long, S. S. (2008). Cellulitis and superficial hand infections. In L. K. Pickering & C. G. Prober (Eds.), *Principles and practice of pediatric infectious disease* (3rd ed.). Retrieved from http://www.mdconsult.com/das/book/body/187327964-17/963263349/1679/76.html#4-u1.0-B978-0-443-06687-0..50075-8–cesec12_1553

Butler, K. H. (2009). Incision and drainage. In J. R. Roberts & J. R. Hedges (Eds.), *Clinical procedures in emergency medicine* (5th ed., pp. 681–685). Philadelphia: Saunders Elsevier.

Clark, D. C. (2003). Common acute hand infections. *American Family Physician, 68*(11), 2167–2176.

Habif, T. P. (2009). Nail diseases. In *Clinical dermatology: A color guide to diagnosis and treatment* (5th ed.). Retrieved from http://www.mdconsult.com/book/player/book.do?method=display&type=bookPage&decorator=header&eid=4-u1.0-B978-0-7234-3541-9..00034-1–s0125&displayedEid=4-u1.0-B978-0-7234-3541-9..00034-1–s0140&uniq=187327964&isbn=978-0-7234-3541-9&sid=963269025.

Lyn, E. T., & Mailhot, T. (2010). Hand: Infection of the hand. *Rosen's Emergency Medicine* (7th ed.). Retrieved from http://www.mdconsult.com/book/player/book.do?method=display&type=bookPage&decorator=header&eid=4-u1.0-B978-0-323-05472-0..X0001-1&uniq=187327964&isbn=978-0-323-05472-0&sid=963266130#lpState=open&lpTab=contentsTab&content=4-u1.0-B978-0-323-05472-0..00047–st0495%3Bfrom%3Dindex%3Btype%3DbookPage%3Bisbn%3D978-0-323-05472-0.

Mostaghimi, L. (2010). Diseases of the skin: Diseases of the nails. In E. T. Bope, R. E. Rakel, & R. D. Kellerman (Eds.), *Conn's current therapy 2010* (1st ed.). Retrieved from http://www.mdconsult.com/book/player/book.do?method=display&type=bookPage&decorator=header&eid=4-u1.0-B978-1-4160-6642-2..00013-2–s0845&uniq=187327964&isbn=978-1-4160-6642-2&sid=963240480

Rockwell, P. G. (2001). Acute and chronic paronychia. *American Family Physician, 63*(6), 1113–1116

Wright, P. E. (2008). Hand infections: Paronychia. In S. T. Canale & J. H. Beaty (Eds.), *Campbell's operative orthopaedics* (11th ed.). Retrieved from http://www.mdconsult.com/das/book/body/187327964-19/963269025/1584/577.html#4-u1.0-B978-0-323-03329-9..50078-7–cesec3_4075

19

Procedures for Treating Felons

Theresa M. Campo

BACKGROUND

A felon is an infection that involves the pulp of the distal finger or thumb. The finger pulp or pad is made up of numerous small compartments that are divided by fibrous septa running from the bone to the skin. The compartments contain eccrine sweat glands and fat globules, which are possible modes of bacterial invasion.

Felons are commonly caused by trauma or a foreign body, such as a splinter, thorn, and so on. An untreated paronychia can develop into a felon. *Staphylococcus aureus*, including methicillin-resistant *S. aureus* (MRSA), is the most common bacteria. However, a mixed infection with staph and strep, as well as a gram-negative infection can occur.

Infection and inflammation can cause an increase in pressure within the compartments and can lead to ischemia and tissue necrosis. Bacteria can invade the periosteum, which can lead to osteomyelitis and can also innervate the flexor tendon sheath.

Complications can develop if the felon is not treated or failure of therapy occurs. Possible complications include osteomyelitis, soft tissue or bone necrosis, septic arthritis of the distal interphalyngeal joint, and flexor tenosynovitis.

PATIENT PRESENTATION

- Rapid onset of pain
  - Continuous and throbbing
- Swelling to distal finger pad
  - Does not extend proximal to distal interphalyngeal joint space
- Redness
- Firmness
  - Fluctuance may be present early but is usually firm at time of patient presentation

  Note: Decreased pain without intervention can be a sign of extensive necrosis and nerve degeneration.

TREATMENT

The definitive treatment for a felon is incision and drainage. Antibiotics alone can be used for minor cellulitis, but are often not curative. Treatment plans should include tetanus prophylaxis, warm compresses or soaks, and elevation. Radiographs should be considered to rule out a foreign body and osteomyelitis. Oral antibiotics should be considered and given based on current recommendations in your region.

Most felons can be effectively managed with a simple incision procedure. The techniques of a "hockey stick" or "fish mouth" incision are not advocated due to the risk of complications; no differences in healing have been found. Careful attention must be paid when incising a felon because of the potential for injury of the tendons, nerves, and vasculature. Incisions should not be performed on the radial aspects of the index finger or the ulnar surface of the thumb or little finger.

SPECIAL CONSIDERATIONS

■ Diabetics
■ Immunocompromised

PROCEDURE PREPARATION

■ Absorbent pads
■ Skin cleanser
■ Lidocaine 1% or 2% with epinephrine (bupivacaine is another option because of its longer duration of action)
■ 10-mL syringe
■ 25-gauge needle for injection of lidocaine
■ No. 11 or No. 15 scalpel blade with handle
■ Scissors
■ Culture swab
■ Normal saline solution
■ Large syringe (20-, 30-, or 35-mL)
■ Gauze pads
■ Kling or gauze for wrapping
■ Tape

Note: Pre-made suture kits usually have the instruments and equipment used in this procedure. Check with your institution for kit contents. Please see Chapter 14 for common contents

PROCEDURE

■ Cleanse the skin using a circular motion to free debris and bacteria
■ Place an absorbent protective pad under the treatment area
■ Drape the patient to maintain a clean area
■ Sterile technique is required for this procedure to prevent extension of the infection
■ Digital block anesthesia should be performed (see Chapter 7)
■ Apply a Penrose drain to the base of the finger to give a bloodless field

Simple Lateral Incision

■ Using either the No. 11 or No. 15 blade scalpel, make an incision at the point of maximum fluctuance (Figure 19.1)
  ■ Incision should be lateral
  ■ Avoid the center or midline finger pad as this may cause increased scarring and pain

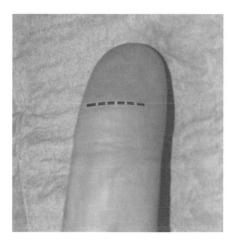

FIGURE 19.1 Felon—Simple lateral incision.

Transverse Incision

■ Make an incision transversely through the point of maximum fluctuance (Figure 19.2)
  ■ Avoid the digital nerves

Longitudinal Incision

■ Longitudinal incision made through the fat pad (Figure 19.3)
  ■ Do not extend past the distal interphalyngeal crease to avoid flexor tendon damage
  ■ This technique should be avoided unless absolutely necessary because of the sensitivity of the fat pad
■ Bluntly dissect the subcutaneous tissue to break up the loculations with a hemostat
■ Investigate, evaluate, and remove foreign bodies
■ Remove any necrotic tissue
■ Irrigate the wound with sterile normal saline and a 20-mL to 30-mL syringe only
  ■ Do not use high pressure irrigation as it may push bacteria onto the tendon sheath and extend the infection into the distal interphalyngeal joint
■ Insert packing into the wound
  ■ Usually only requires a wick (small piece of packing)
■ Dress the wound with gauze and Kling

Alternate Procedure—Through-and-Through Incision

■ A second incision can be made similarly to the first to allow a "through-and-through" incision (Figure 19.4)
■ Place gauze in the first incision
■ Grasp the gauze through the second incision and pull through
■ Trim the gauze close to the finger
■ Dress the wound with gauze and Kling
■ Finger splint may be applied

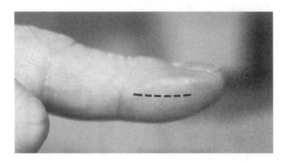

FIGURE 19.2 Felon—Transverse incision.

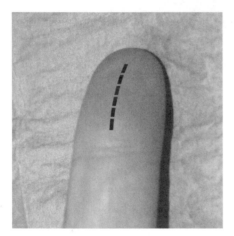

FIGURE 19.3 Felon—Longitudinal incision.

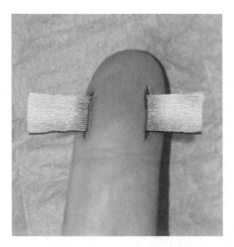

FIGURE 19.4 Felon—Through-and-through technique.

POSTPROCEDURE CONSIDERATIONS

Pain

■ Instruct the patient to keep the finger elevated, above the level of the heart, to prevent throbbing and pain

EDUCATIONAL POINTS

■ Elevate
■ Warm compresses
■ Packing removal 48 to 72 hours
■ Narcotic analgesia with instructions not to drive or consume alcohol with medication

COMPLICATIONS

■ Extension or recurrence of infection
■ Osteomyelitis
■ Soft tissue necrosis
■ Bone necrosis
■ Nerve damage
■ Heightened sensitivity to the distal finger
■ Scar tissue

Author's Pearls

■ *Premedicate with oral pain medicine if not driving home*
■ *Cutting the finger out of a sterile glove and placing at the base of the finger can be done in place of a Penrose drain*

RESOURCES

Browning, J., Levy, M., & Long, S. S. (2008). Cellulitis and superficial hand infections. In L. K. Pickering & C. G. Prober (Eds.), *Principles and practice of pediatric infectious disease* (3rd ed.). Retrieved from http://www.mdconsult.com/das/book/body/187327964-20/963270106/1584/578.html#4-u1.0-B978-0-323-03329-9..50078-7–cesec7_4079

Clark, D. C. (2003). Common acute hand infections. *American Family Physician, 68*(11), 2167–2176.

Lyn, E. T., & Mailhot, T. (2010). Hand: Infection of the hand. *Rosen's emergency medicine* (7th ed.). Retrieved from http://www.mdconsult.com/book/player/book.do?method=display&type=bookPage&decorator=header&eid=4-u1.0-B978-0-323-05472-0..00047-5–s0705&displayedEid=4-u1.0-B978-0-323-05472-0..00047-5–s0730&uniq=187327964&isbn=978-0-323-05472-0&sid=963271883

Mostaghimi, L. (2010). Diseases of the skin: Diseases of the nails. In E. T. Bope, R. E. Rakel, & R. D. Kellerman (Eds.), *Conn's current therapy 2010* (1st ed.). Retrieved from http://www.mdconsult.com/book/player/book.do?method=display&type=bookPage&decorator=header&eid=4-u1.0-B978-1-4160-6642-2..00013-2–s0845&uniq=187327964&isbn=978-1-4160-6642-2&sid=963240480

Vaughn, G. (2010, March 25). Felon. Retrieved from http://emedicine.medscape.com/article/ 782537-overview and http://emedicine.medscape.com/article/782537-treatment

Wright, P. E. (2008). Hand infections: Paronychia. In S. T. Canale & J. H. Beaty (Eds.), *Campbell's operative orthopaedics* (11th ed.). Retrieved from http://www.mdconsult.com/das/ book/body/187327964-19/963269025/1584/577.html#4-u1.0-B978-0-323-03329-9. 50078-7–cesec3_4075

Abscess Overview

THERESA M. CAMPO

An abscess is the formation and collection of pus that can develop in any region of the body, usually initiated by the breakdown of epidermal defense mechanisms against the normal flora. It can occur by either an inflammatory reaction to an infectious process (bacteria, parasite, or fungus) or less commonly by a foreign body or substance such as a splinter or needle. Abscesses may develop from a blocked sweat or oil gland (sebaceous), from an inflamed hair follicle, or minor break in the skin such as a puncture wound.

The most typical organism causing an abscess is *Staphylococcus aureus*; normally found on the skin, it produces an area of rapidly forming necrosis and large amounts of pus. Group A β-hemolytic streptococcus tends to spread rapidly through the tissue causing erythema, edema, and serous exudate with little or no necrosis. It also has a streaky appearance and is the cause of most cellulitis. In the perirectal area, enteric and/or anaerobic bacteria proliferation is typical. Necrosis and brownish, foul smelling pus is typical of abscess formation and is commonly seen with cellulitis of the surrounding tissue. Combinations of anaerobic and gram-negative organisms have been reported in the literature. Recently, methicillin-resistant *Staphylococcus aureus* has been identified as the source of many abscesses throughout the nation and the world due to the misuse and overuse of antibiotics.

Abscesses form when white blood cells (WBC) move through the walls of the blood vessels into an area with organisms or foreign bodies. The WBCs collect with the damaged tissue, forming pus, which is a build up of fluid, damaged and dead tissue, and organisms, usually bacteria. A pocket forms with the pus and a wall is formed to attempt to block the bacteria from spreading to surrounding tissue or structures initiating an inflammatory response. Occasionally, bacteria escape from the walled-off area and penetrate the blood stream and surrounding tissue or organs.

Most abscesses occur cutaneously and can be found in the extremities (especially axilla), groin and external vagina (bartholin), tailbone (pilonidal), and areas of hair distribution causing a folliculitis, which can then form a furuncle. Abscesses can also occur in the brain, liver, kidneys, lungs, teeth/periodontal, pharynx, and tonsils. Common areas related to a patient's occupation and intravenous drug use can be viewed in Table 20.1.

TABLE 20.1 Factors Leading to Abscess Formation and Location

Factor	Body Area/Location	Cause
Occupation (manual labor)	Arms Hands	Minor trauma
Women	Axilla Groin Submammary	Shaving Constrictive clothing Overgrowth of bacteria

Intravenous drug users
  (may be superficial or deep)
	Upper extremities
	Lower extremities
		Penetration of skin with clean
		  or dirty needles
		Skin popping

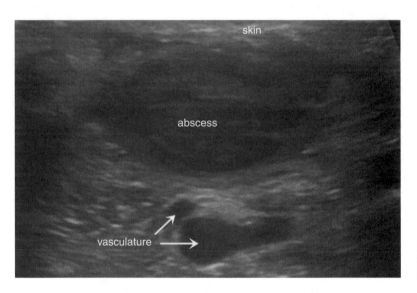

FIGURE 20.1
Ultrasound of
subcutaneous abscess.

Most abscesses can be readily diagnosed based on the physical examination findings of pain, redness, swelling, and the presence of fluctuance. When the physical findings are equivocal, needle aspiration and/or ultrasonography may be performed. The use of ultrasonography is increasing in popularity and can assist in the location and diagnosis of abscess formation, especially in areas with major vessels and organs in close proximity to the affected area. Ultrasonography can easily identify surrounding arteries with the use of the Doppler color setting (Figure 20.1).

RESOURCES

Abrahamian, F. M., Talan, D. A., & Moran, G. J. (2008). Management of skin and soft tissue infections in the emergency department. *Infectious Disease Clinics of North America,* *22*(1), 89–116.

Anderson, D. J., & Kaye, K. S. (2007). Skin and soft tissue infections in older adults. *Clinics in Geriatric Medicine, 23*(3), 595–613.

Butler, K. H. (2010). Incision and drainage. In J. R. Roberts & J. R. Hedges (Eds.), *Clinical procedures in emergency medicine* (5th ed., pp. 657–672). Philadelphia: Saunders Elsevier.

Fitch, M. T., Manthey, D. E., McGinnis, H. D., Nicks, B. A., & Pariyadath, M. (2007). Abscess incision and drainage. *New England Journal of Medicine, 357*(19), e20.

Grimm, L., & Carmody, K. A. (2009, May 20). Bedside ultrasonography, abscess evaluation. Retrieved from http://emedicine.medscape.com/article/1379916-overview & http://emedicine.medscape.com/article/1379916-treatment

Hammond, S. P., & Baden, L. R. (2008). Management of skin and soft-tissue infection—Polling results. *New England Journal of Medicine, 359*(19), e20.

Meislin, H. W., & Guisto, J .A. (2009). Soft tissue infections. In J. A. Marx, R. Hockberger, & R. Walls (Eds.), *Rosen's emergency medicine* (7th ed.). Retrieved from http://www.mdconsult.com/book/player/book.do?method=display&type=bookPage&decorator=header&eid=4-u1.0-B978-0-323-05472-0..00135-3–s0325&uniq=190201654&isbn=978-0-323-05472-0&sid=970896658

Rogers, R. L., & Perkins, J. (2006). Skin and soft tissue infections. *Primary Care Clinical Office Practice, 33*(3), 697–710.

Singer, A. J., & Dagum, A. B. (2008). Current management of acute cutaneous wounds. *New England Journal of Medicine, 359*(10), 1037–1046.

21

Procedure for Incision and Drainage of Subcutaneous Abscess

Theresa M. Campo

BACKGROUND

Abscesses most commonly occur in the following areas:

- Extremities (especially axilla)
- Areas of hair distribution (folliculitis, furuncle)
- Neck
- Buttocks

PATIENT PRESENTATION

- Red, raised, painful lump
- Warmth
- Firm and/or fluctuant (fluid filled, feels like a ripe piece of fruit)
- Pointing with pustule
- Lymphangitis
- Lymphadenopathy
- Localized or extensive cellulitis
- Fever

TREATMENT

Incision and drainage is considered to be the definitive treatment for cutaneous abscesses. Abscesses without cellulitis can be effectively treated with incision and drainage alone and may not require antibiotic treatment. Deep seated abscesses or abscesses over major vessels or structures can be investigated further using ultrasonography or CT scanning. Abscesses found within or extending into the abdominal cavity, thoracic cavity, brain, and other deep tissue can be incised using guided imaging.

Abscesses that are fluctuant and draining can develop a chronic nonhealing sinus that may require surgical excision. Cultures should be obtained when incising any abscess to determine the offending organism(s), especially methicillin-resistant *Staphylococcus aureus*. Small lesions, usually less than 5 mm, can be treated effectively with warm compresses and either topical or systemic antibiotics based on the severity and location of the infection. Larger abscesses should be incised and drained, with packing removal in 24 to 48 hours of placement. Any abscess with pus formation, whether firm or fluctuant, should be incised and drained. Antibiotic treatment alone does not adequately treat loculated collections of pus and infection. Incisions should be liberal to allow for break up of loculations and appropriate drainage of the purulent material. Accompanying cellulitis should be treated empirically based on the common organisms found in the region (i.e., methicillin-resistant *Staphylococcus aureus* [MRSA]). Modifications to treatment can be made once culture results are reported.

Some abscesses located at cosmetically important areas and not significant on physical examination can be evacuated by needle aspiration as long as the purulent material is not too thick for drainage. Large abscesses may require a rubber drain to be placed. All abscesses should be evaluated and treated independently, with careful consideration given to the patient's past and current medical history, family history, and current trends of bacterial organism invasion in the treatment area.

CONTRAINDICATIONS AND RELATIVE CONTRAINDICATIONS

- Abscesses that lie in close proximity to major vessel
  - Location and nature of abscess should be confirmed with needle aspiration, ultrasonography, or CT scan
- Hand abscesses involving the palmer aspect and with passive range of motion pain should be referred immediately to a hand specialist for evaluation and treatment
  - Increased severity of infection occurs because the flexor tendon has a sheath of synovial fluid and the extensor tendon does not

SPECIAL CONSIDERATIONS

- Pediatric patient
  - Conscious sedation may be necessary for deep-seated or difficult-to-manage areas due to movement or severity
  - Each case should be considered independently
- General anesthesia
  - May be required for abscesses located in the perirectal, supralevator, ischiorectal areas, and those that are deep-seated or in the area of major vessels or over bony prominences
- Abscesses located in the palmer aspect of the hand should be referred to a hand specialist to avoid tendon injury or neurovascular compromise
- Abscesses located on the face, particularly the nasolabial fold, may drain into the sphenoid sinus causing cavernous sinus thrombosis
- Immunocompromised and comorbidities
  - Abscesses in organ transplant, HIV, AIDS, diabetes, and/or cancer patients should be treated more aggressively and with a lower index of suspicion for abscess and infection
  - Patients with immunosuppression may not present with classic signs and symptoms of abscess formation as they may lack the host defense and release of cytokines producing the inflammatory reaction. They may only present with a low grade fever or malaise. Atypical bacterial organisms and fungus are more common in this population
- Intravenous (IV) drug use

- Patients with multiple abscesses or abscesses on the arms and antecubital fossa or dorsal aspect of the hand should be questioned for IV drug use, and treated more aggressively for atypical organisms and fungus
- Pregnancy
  - Patients who are pregnant should be treated with antibiotics that are considered safe in pregnancy
- Artificial heart valves and prosthetic joints
  - Prophylaxis based on the current American Heart Association/American College of Cardiology guidelines
  - The timing of the procedure may need to be reconsidered to help prevent endo-carditis in this group of patients
  - Consultation with a specialist is recommended

PROCEDURE PREPARATION

- Protective gown, gloves, and goggles—abscess contents are under pressure
- Drape
- Skin cleanser
- Lidocaine 1% or 2% with epinephrine (bupivacaine is another option due to its longer duration of action)
- 20- or 35-mL syringe for irrigation
- 10-mL syringe
- 25-Gauge needle for injection of lidocaine
- No. 11 or No. 15 scalpel blade with handle
- Hemostat and scissors
- Culture swab
- Normal saline solution
- Plain or iodoform 1/4, 1/2, or 1 inch depending upon the size and depth of the abscess
- Gauze pads
- Kling or gauze for wrapping
- Tape

PROCEDURE

- Cleanse the skin using a circular motion to free debris and bacteria
- Place an absorbent protective pad under the treatment area
- Drape the patient to maintain a clean area as well as to protect the patient's privacy
- Strict sterile technique is not required for this procedure. However, because of the era of resistance, sterile technique should be used whenever possible

Infiltration

- Anesthetize the top of the wound inserting a 25-gauge needle just under and parallel to the surface of the skin
- Inject the anesthetic gently, into the intradermal layer, until the area is large enough for incision (Figure 21.1). Field block anesthesia can be used for larger abscesses. See Chapter 5.
- You will notice blanching of the skin

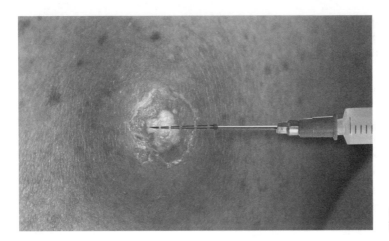

FIGURE 21.1 Intradermal infiltration of abscess.

Incision

- Make a liberal incision directly over the center of the abscess with a No. 11 or No. 15 scalpel making sure to cut through the skin and into the cavity of the abscess (Figure 21.2)
  - Direct, firm pressure should be used when making the incision
- Be careful not to puncture through the back end of the abscess wall because this can cause excessive bleeding
- Extend the incision to allow for adequate drainage of pus and enough room for wound dissection
- Attention should be given to the skin tension lines; these should be followed whenever possible for the best cosmetic outcome
- Allow the pus to drain freely and apply pressure to the area to assist with expression of pus and abscess contents
- With a culture swab, swab the *inside* of the abscess—not the drainage (Figure 21.3)

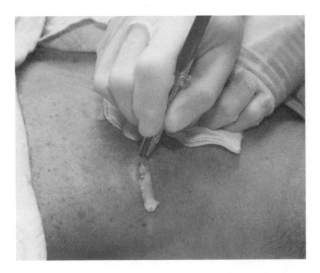

FIGURE 21.2 Incising an abscess.

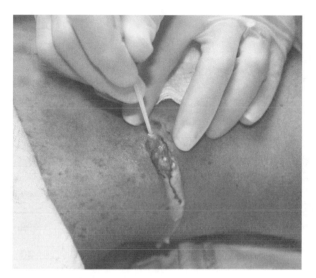

FIGURE 21.3 Obtaining a culture swab.

- Perform a blunt dissection with a curved hemostat in a circular motion to break up loculations (Figure 21.4)
- Never use a gloved finger especially when a foreign body is suspected
- Irrigate the abscess liberally with normal saline (Figure 21.5)
- Insert iodoform or plain packing into the cavity (Figure 21.6)
- Place a sufficient amount of packing into the cavity, making certain not to over pack the wound causing pressure necrosis, which causes ischemia and death to the surrounding tissue
- Apply a gauze dressing to help collect any drainage

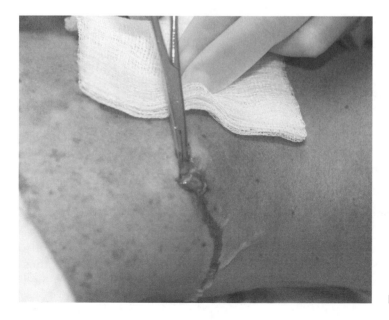

FIGURE 21.4 Blunt dissection.

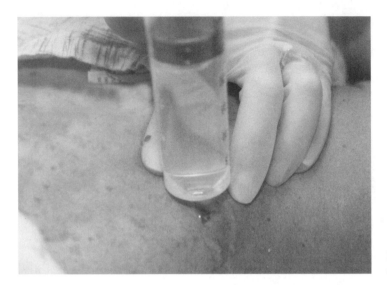

FIGURE 21.5 Irrigation of an abscess cavity.

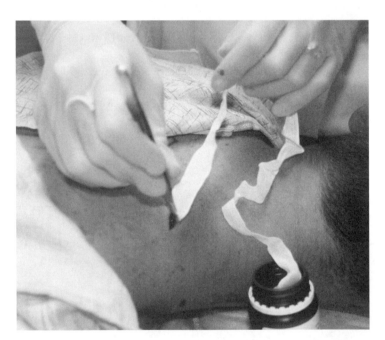

FIGURE 21.6 Insertion of packing.

■ Tetanus immunization should be up to date
■ Abscesses should not be sutured closed

POSTPROCEDURE CONSIDERATIONS

Pain

The contents of the abscess are acidotic and can decrease the efficacy of the anesthetic. Performance of a field block (see Chapter 5) and administering oral pain medicine can help reduce the pain.

Drainage

- If there is little or no drainage from the abscess, consider a deeper and/or wider incision.
- If sebaceous material is extracted from the site and there is little or no pus, proceed with the procedure as described previously.

Antibiotic Therapy

Successful incision and drainage of abscesses do not require antibiotic therapy in healthy individuals unless the abscess is accompanied by cellulitis. However, patients who are immunocompromised, diabetic, or IV drug users should be considered for antibiotic treatment. It has been speculated that abscesses caused by community-acquired MRSA do not need antibiotic therapy. However, there is few data to support this at this time.

EDUCATIONAL POINTS

- Packing should be changed if persistent drainage is present; otherwise removal within 48 hours of placement is recommended during follow-up with a provider
- Stress the importance of follow-up
- Risks and benefits of antibiotics and pain medicine
- Area should not get wet until packing is removed
- Healing occurs through tissue granulation from the base of the wound
- Proper hygiene and hand washing are effective against recurrence and spread of infection

COMPLICATIONS

- Progression of infection to surrounding tissue causing cellulitis, lymphangitis, and/or fever should be treated with antibiotic therapy
- Recurrence of the abscess necessitates consideration of risk factors or abnormalities, including foreign body, cancer, staph colonization, and immunologic disorders

---

AUTHOR'S PEARLS

- *Fluctuance can be described to patients as a piece of ripe or over-ripe fruit such as a peach*
- *Premedicating with oral analgesia helps to make the procedure more tolerable*
- *Peripads can be used for abscesses in the groin or buttocks or areas that are difficult to dress with tape or wrapping gauze*
- *Patients presenting with pus should not leave with pus*

RESOURCES

Abrahamian, F. M., Talan, D. A., & Moran, G. J. (2008). Management of skin and soft tissue infections in the emergency department. *Infectious Disease Clinics of North America, 22*(1), 89–116.

Anderson, D. J., & Kaye, K. S. (2007). Skin and soft tissue infections in older adults. *Clinics in Geriatric Medicine, 23*(3), 595–613.

Butler, K. H. (2010). Incision and drainage. In J. R. Roberts & J. R. Hedges (Eds.), *Clinical procedures in emergency medicine* (5th ed., pp. 657–672). Philadelphia: Saunders Elsevier.

Fitch, M. T., Manthey, D. E., McGinnis, H. D., Nicks, B. A., & Pariyadath, M. (2007). Abscess incision and drainage. *New England Journal of Medicine, 357*(19), e20.

Grimm, L., & Carmody, K. A. (2009, May 20). Bedside ultrasonography, abscess evaluation. Retrieved from http://emedicine.medscape.com/article/1379916-overview & http://emedicine.medscape.com/article/1379916-treatment

Hammond, S. P., & Baden, L. R. (2008). Management of skin and soft-tissue infection— Polling results. *New England Journal of Medicine, 359*(19), e20.

Meislin, H. W., & Guisto, J. A. (2009). Soft tissue infections. In J. A. Marx, R. Hockberger, & R. Walls (Eds.), *Rosen's emergency medicine* (7th ed.). Retrieved from http://www.mdconsult.com/book/player/book.do?method=display&type=bookPage&decorator=header&eid=4-u1.0-B978-0-323-05472-0..00135-3–s0325&uniq=190201654&isbn=978-0-323-05472-0&sid=970896658

Rogers, R. L., & Perkins, J. (2006). Skin and soft tissue infections. *Primary Care Clinical Office Practice, 33*(3), 697–710.

Singer, A. J., & Dagum, A. B. (2008). Current management of acute cutaneous wounds. *New England Journal of Medicine, 359*(10), 1037–1046.

Procedure for Managing Pilonidal Cyst/Abscess

THERESA M. CAMPO

BACKGROUND

The term pilonidal has its origins from the Latin terms "pilus" meaning hair and "nidus" meaning nest. Pilonidal abscesses were originally thought to be congenital and caused by remnants of caudal segments, hair, and other dermal debris. However, during World War II, there was an insurgence of soldiers who were jeep drivers that suffered from pilonidal abscesses. It was postulated that the cysts could be caused by repetitive trauma. The most recent theory on the development of pilonidal abscesses is that a foreign body reaction occurs. Microtrauma causes the epithelium to line the cavity, which in turn causes that occlusion that prevents drainage. Hair follicle enlargement then causes an inflammatory response and edema. The increased pressure causes the spreading of purulent material to the surrounding subcutaneous tissue, thus promoting abscess formation. These abscesses can be quite large and are found in the gluteal fold overlying the coccyx. See Figure 22.1 to visualize a pilonidal abscess.

 Staphylococcus aureus, anaerobic cocci, aerobic, and anaerobic organisms cause abscess formation. Abscesses are more prevalent in men than in women. They tend to be familial and occur in persons with sitting occupations and obesity.

PATIENT PRESENTATION

- Sinus tract or "pit" sacrococcygeal region
- Tenderness to palpation
- Back pain
- Fluctuance
- Warmth
- Purulent discharge
- Localized or extensive cellulitis
- Fever

TREATMENT

The goal of treatment for pilonidal abscess is to fully remove the internalized material (i.e., hair, keratin, and cellular debris). Simple incision and drainage can be performed to treat the acute fluctuant abscess until surgical excision of the internalized

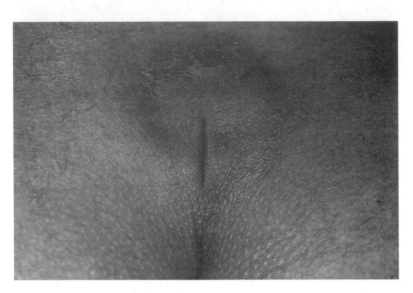

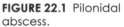

FIGURE 22.1 Pilonidal abscess.

material can be done. Pilonidal abscesses have a varied recurrence rate that can be as high as 90%. Even with surgical excision, 20% to 40% may recur. A flared-end de Pezzer catheter may be used for an extended period of time to allow for granulation and closure of chronic sinus. Simple incision and drainage of pilonidal abscess will be the focus of this chapter.

CONTRAINDICATIONS AND RELATIVE CONTRAINDICATIONS

- Immunocompromised

SPECIAL CONSIDERATIONS

- Immunocompromised
- Diabetic
- Cancer
- HIV-positive patient
- Pregnancy
- Pediatric and elderly patients
- Comorbidities
- Prosthetic heart valves
- Prosthetic joints

PROCEDURE PREPARATION

- Protective gown, gloves, and goggles—abscess contents are under pressure
- Drape
- Skin cleanser
- Lidocaine 1% or 2% with epinephrine (bupivacaine is another option because of its longer duration of action)
- 20- or 35-mL syringe for irrigation
- 10-mL syringe

- 25-gauge needle for injection of lidocaine
- No. 11 or No. 15 scalpel blade with handle
- Hemostat and scissors
- Culture swab
- Normal saline solution
- Suture kit
- Plain or iodoform 1/4, 1/2, or 1 inch depending upon the size and depth of the abscess
- Gauze pads
- Kling or gauze for wrapping
- Tape

PROCEDURE

- Cleanse the skin using a circular motion to free debris and bacteria
- Place an absorbent protective pad under the treatment area
- Drape the patient to maintain a clean area as well as to protect the patient's privacy
- Strict sterile technique is not required for this procedure. However, because of the era of resistance, sterile technique should be used whenever possible

Note: Figures illustrating the following procedural steps appear in Chapter 21.

Infiltration

- Anesthetize the top of the wound inserting a 25-gauge needle just under and parallel to the surface of the skin
- Inject the anesthetic gently into the indradermal layer, until the area is large enough for incision
- You will notice blanching of the skin.

Incision

- Make a liberal incision directly over the center of the abscess with a No. 11 or No. 15 scalpel making sure to cut through the skin and into the cavity of the abscess
  - Direct, firm pressure should be used when making the incision
- Be careful not to puncture through the back end of the abscess wall because this can cause excessive bleeding
- Extend the incision to allow for adequate drainage of pus and enough room for wound dissection
- Attention should be given to the skin tension lines; these should be followed whenever possible for the best cosmetic outcome
- Allow the pus to drain freely and apply pressure to the area to assist with expression of pus and abscess contents
- With a culture swab, swab the inside of the abscess—not the drainage (Figure 21.3)
- Perform a blunt dissection with a curved hemostat in a circular motion to break up loculations
- Never use a gloved finger especially when a foreign body is suspected
- Irrigate the abscess liberally with normal saline

■ Insert iodoform or plain packing into the cavity
■ Place a sufficient amount of packing into the cavity making certain not to over pack the wound causing pressure necrosis, which causes ischemia and death to the surrounding tissue
■ Apply a gauze dressing to help collect any drainage
■ Tetanus immunization should be up to date
■ Abscesses should not be sutured closed

POSTPROCEDURE CONSIDERATIONS

Pain

■ The contents of the abscess are acidotic and can decrease the efficacy of the anesthetic
■ Performance of a field block and administering oral pain medicine can help reduce the pain

Drainage

■ If little or no drainage from the abscess, consider a deeper and/or wider incision
■ If sebaceous material is extracted from the site and there is little or no pus, proceed with the procedure as described previously

Antibiotic Therapy

■ Successful incision and drainage of abscesses do not require antibiotic therapy in healthy individuals unless the abscess is accompanied by cellulitis
■ Patients who are immunocompromised, diabetic, or IV drug users should be considered for antibiotic treatment
■ It has been speculated that abscesses caused by community-acquired methicillin-resistant *Staphylococcus aureus* (MRSA) do not need antibiotic therapy. However, there is few data to support this at this time

EDUCATIONAL POINTS

■ Packing should be changed if persistent drainage is present, otherwise removal within 48 hours of placement is recommended during follow-up with a provider
■ Stress the importance of follow-up
■ Risks and benefits of antibiotics and pain medicine
■ Area should not get wet until the packing is removed
■ Healing occurs through tissue granulation from the base of the wound
■ Proper hygiene and hand washing is effective against recurrence and spread of infection
■ The use of a donut pillow will help to reduce the pressure on the affected area

COMPLICATIONS

■ Progression of infection to surrounding tissue causing cellulitis, lymphangitis, and/or fever should be treated with antibiotic therapy
■ Recurrence of the abscess necessitates consideration of risk factors or abnormalities including foreign body, cancer, staph colonization, and immunologic disorders

AUTHOR'S PEARLS

- *Instruct patients who have sitting occupations to take frequent breaks or use donut pillows to reduce the pressure on the coccyx area*
- *Don't forget to medicate for pain. This can be a painful experience*

RESOURCES

Butler, K. H. (2010). Incision and drainage. In J. R. Roberts & J. R. Hedges (Eds.), *Clinical procedures in emergency medicine* (5th ed., pp. 677–679). Philadelphia: Saunders Elsevier.

Coates, W. C. (2009). Disorders of the anorectum. In J. A. Marx, R. Hockberger, & R. Walls (Eds.), *Rosen's emergency medicine* (7th ed.). Retrieved from http://www.mdconsult.com/book/player/book.do?method=display&type=bookPage&decorator=header&eid=4-u1.0-B978-0-323-05472-0..00094-3–s0180&uniq=190201654&isbn=978-0-323-05472-0&sid=970898882

Fazeli, M. S., Ghavami, M., & Lebaschi, A. H. (2006). Comparison of outcomes in z plasty and delayed healing by secondary intention of the wound after excision of the sacral pilonidal sinus: Results of a randomized, clinical trial. *Diseases of the Colon and Rectum, 49*(12), 1831–1836.

Lanigan, M. D. (2009, August 6). Pilonidal cyst and sinus. Retrieved from http://emedicine.medscape.com/article/788127-overview & http://emedicine.medscape.com/article/788127-treatment

Lee, P. J., Raniga, S., Biyani, D. K., Watson, A. J., Faragher, I. G., & Frizelli, F. A. (2008). Sacrococcygeal pilonidal disease. *Colorectal Disease, 10*(7), 639–650.

Tajirian, T., Lee, J. L., & Abbas, M. A. (2007). Is wide local excision for pilonidal disease still justified? *The American Surgeon, 73*(10), 1075–1078.

Procedure for Managing Bartholin Abscess

Theresa M. Campo

BACKGROUND

The Bartholin gland is a secretory organ approximately the size of a pea. It is located at the posterior introitus bilaterally at 5 and 7 o'clock on each side of the vestibule of the vagina. This gland drains through ducts that empty into the vestibule. It maintains the moisture of the vaginal mucosa. Obstruction of the duct may result in the formation of a cyst or abscess when there is retention of secretions, which causes the duct to dilate. A Bartholin abscess can be a common problem in women of reproductive age. It is distinguishable from a cyst in that an abscess produces a rapid onset of swelling and pain in the vulvar area. Cysts are often asymptomatic in nature. Figure 23.1 shows a Bartholin gland abscess.

MOST COMMON ORGANISMS

Aerobic

- *Neisseria gonorrhoeae*
- *Staphylococcus aureus*
- *Streptococcus faecalis*
- *Escherichia coli*
- *Pseudomonas aeruginosa*
- *Chlamydia trachomatis*

Anaerobic

- *Bacteroides fragilis*
- *Clostridium perfringens*
- *Peptostreptococcus* species
- *Fusobacterium* species

PATIENT PRESENTATION

- Acute unilateral swelling of labia minora
- Pain with walking and sitting
- Exquisitely tender mass—grape size
- Dyspareunia—painful intercourse
- Fluctuant

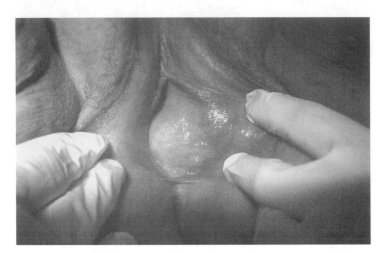

FIGURE 23.1 Bartholin abscess.

- Erythema
- Spontaneous rupture with purulent drainage
- Localized cellulitis
- Systemic infection is not common with this type of abscess

TREATMENT

Simple incision and drainage with or without insertion of a word catheter is the initial treatment for a Bartholin abscess. Removal of the gland or marsupalization may be performed if recurrence is an issue but is not often considered for initial treatment. The goal of treatment is drainage of the abscess contents, prevention of fluid reaccumulation, and pain relief. Bartholin abscesses are painful, and patient comfort during the incision and drainage should be a priority.

Simple incision and drainage with and without insertion of a word catheter will be covered in this chapter. Whenever a word catheter is available, it should be used for both initial and long-term treatment, as it may obviate the need for marsupalization. The word catheter allows for epithelialization to occur.

CONTRAINDICATIONS AND RELATIVE CONTRAINDICATIONS

Complex or recurrent abscesses may require general anesthesia for removal of the Bartholin gland.

SPECIAL CONSIDERATIONS

- Immunocompromised
- Diabetic
- Cancer
- HIV-positive
- Pregnancy

PROCEDURE PREPARATION

- Protective gown, gloves, and goggles—abscess contents are under pressure

- Absorbent pad
- Drape
- Skin cleanser
- Lidocaine 1% (bupivacaine is another option due to its longer duration of action)
- 20- or 35-mL syringe for irrigation
- 10-mL syringe
- 25-gauge needle for injection of lidocaine
- No. 11 or No. 15 scalpel blade with handle
- Hemostat, scissors
- Culture swab
- Normal saline solution
- Plain or iodoform 1/4, 1/2, or 1 inch depending on size and depth of abscess
- Peri-pad

PROCEDURE

- Cleanse the skin using a circular motion to free debris and bacteria
- Place an absorbent protective pad under the treatment area
- Place the patient in the lithotomy position
- Drape the patient to maintain a clean area as well as to protect the patient's privacy
- Strict sterile technique is not required for this procedure. However, due to the era of resistance, sterile technique should be used whenever possible

Infiltration

- Insert a 25-gauge needle into the subcutaneous layer of the labia minora just under the mucosa
- Infiltrate the area with lidocaine 1% (1–3 mL)

Incision

- Make a small incision along the medial mucosa, not the skin, with a No. 11 scalpel
- Use the tip of the scalpel or a hemostat to puncture the abscess cavity
- Make an incision that is large enough to allow for proper drainage of fluid contents (Figure 23.2)
- Be careful not to puncture through the back end of the abscess wall, as this can cause excessive bleeding
- Allow the pus to drain freely; apply pressure to the area to assist with expression of pus and abscess contents
- With a culture swab, swab the inside of the abscess; not the drainage
- Never use a gloved finger especially when a foreign body is suspected
- Perform a blunt dissection with a curved hemostat in a circular motion to break up loculations
- Irrigate the abscess liberally with normal saline
- Insert iodoform or plain packing into the cavity
- Place a sufficient amount of packing into the cavity making certain not to over pack the wound causing pressure necrosis, which causes ischemia and death to the surrounding tissue

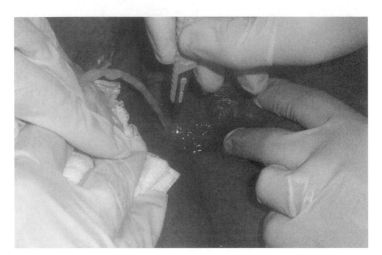

FIGURE 23.2 Incising a Bartholin abscess.

Insertion of a Word Catheter

■ Make the incision large enough to fit the deflated word catheter but small enough to hold the inflated balloon of the catheter in place
■ Place the deflated catheter inside the cavity (Figure 23.3)
■ Using a 25-gauge needle, instill 2- to 4-mL of water into the stopper
■ Place the free end of the catheter into the vagina
■ The catheter should remain in place for 2 to 4 weeks
■ Apply a gauze dressing to help collect any drainage
■ Tetanus immunization should be up to date
■ Abscesses should not be sutured closed

POSTPROCEDURE CONSIDERATIONS

Incising the Abscess

■ Failure to obtain pus or to feel a "pop" after the small incision is made in the mucosa and the cavity is punctured may indicate a failed procedure
■ "Skewer" the abscess onto a hemostat by stabilizing the abscess between the thumb and index finger first

Persistent Pain

■ Too much fluid accumulation after packing or word catheter insertion
■ Make a larger incision to facilitate proper drainage, then reinsert packing
■ Consider the marsupalization procedure

Word Catheter Falls Out

■ Incision too big to hold catheter in place—consider using packing
■ Word catheter reinsertion can be done if it falls out before the 2- to 4-week time period

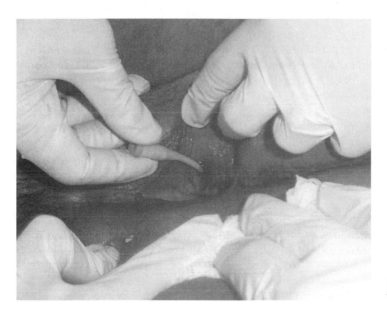

FIGURE 23.3 Insertion of word catheter.

EDUCATIONAL POINTS

- Packing should be changed if persistent drainage is present, otherwise removal within 48 hours of placement is recommended during follow-up with a provider
- Stress the importance of follow-up
- Risks and benefits of antibiotics and pain medicine
- Area should not get wet until the packing is removed
- Area can get wet if word catheter inserted
- Word catheter should ideally remain in place for 2 to 4 weeks but may fall out within 1 week
- Sexual intercourse is not contraindicated with a word catheter insertion

COMPLICATIONS

- Bleeding
- Progressive infection, cellulitis, and sepsis
- Recurrence

AUTHOR'S PEARLS

- *Don't forget to medicate for pain. This can be a painful experience*
- *Use a peri-pad to protect clothing from drainage*
- *Alert patients of the foul odor that may emanate from the abscess once it is incised. Use peppermint oil or air freshener before the procedure*
- *A fracture bedpan under the patient's buttocks can assist with drainage. Some abscess drain a lot of fluid and patients won't want to lie in it*

RESOURCES

Birnbauer, D. M., & Anderegg, C. (2009). Sexually transmitted diseases. In J. A. Marx, R. Hockberger, & R. Walls (Eds.), *Rosen's emergency medicine* (7th ed.). Retrieved from http://www.mdconsult.com/book/player/book.do?method=display&type=bookPage& decorator=header&eid=4-u1.0-B978-0-323-05472-0..00096-7–s0035&uniq=190201654& isbn=978-0-323-05472-0&sid=970896658#lpState=open&lpTab=contentsTab&content= 4-u1.0-B978-0-323-05472-0..00096-7–s0035%3Bfrom%3Dtoc%3Btype%3DbookPage% 3Bisbn%3D978-0-323-05472-0

Butler, K. H. (2010). Incision and drainage. In J. R. Roberts & J. R. Hedges (Eds.), *Clinical procedures in emergency medicine* (5th ed., pp. 674–677). Philadelphia: Saunders Elsevier.

Hill, D. A., & Lense, J. J. (1998). Office management of Bartholin gland cysts and abscesses. *American Family Physician*. Retrieved from http://www.aafp.org/afp/980401ap/hill.html

Meislin, H. W., & Guisto, J. A. (2009). Soft tissue infections. In J. A. Marx, R. Hockberger, & R. Walls (Eds.), *Rosen's emergency medicine* (7th ed.). Retrieved from http://www.mdconsult. com/book/player/book.do?method=display&type=bookPage&decorator=header&eid= 4-u1.0-B978-0-323-05472-0..00135-3–s0325&uniq=190201654&isbn=978-0-323-05472- 0&sid=970896658

Omole, F., Simmons, B. J., & Hacker, Y. (2003). Management of Bartholin duct cyst and gland abscess. *American Family Physician 68(1)*, 135–140.

Patil, S., Sultan, A. H., & Thaker, R. (2007). Bartholin's cysts and abscesses. *Journal of Obstetrics and Gynaecology 27(3)*, 241–245.

Peibert, J. F. (2003). Genital chlamydial infections. *The New England journal of Medicine 349(25)*, 2424–2430.

Schecter, J. C., & Quinn, A. (2009). Bartholin gland disease. Retrieved from http://emedicine. medscape.com/article/777112-overview & http://emedicine.medscape.com/article/777112- treatment

Schlamovitz, G. Z. (2009). Drainage, Bartholin abscess. Retrieved from http://emedicine. medscape.com/article/80260-overview & http://emedicine.medscape.com/article/80260- treatment

Eye Examination

LARRY ISAACS

BACKGROUND

Before the eye examination, a history and timing of the complaint is important. Obtain pertinent ophthalmologic history such as surgeries, prescription drop use, or corrective glasses/contact lens use. If a chemical injury to the eye has occurred, any detailed examination should occur after copious irrigation with water or saline of the affected eye(s).

GENERAL EYE EXAMINATION

Visual Acuity

Corrected visual acuity should be documented. If vision is severely affected, counting fingers and light perception are two measures for documenting severely impaired vision. One can use an index card with a pinhole if the patient does not have his/her glasses.

External Exam

Begin with lids/lashes looking for swelling, discharge (matted lashes), and lacerations. Notice any proptosis, ptosis, or asymmetry. Any lid laceration on the medial third of the lid gives risk of lacrimal duct injury and should be considered for repair by an ophthalmologist.

Extraocular Movements

Cranial nerves III, IV, and VI control eye movements; cranial nerve III also controls pupillary constriction and lid elevation. Have the patient move his/her eyes in all directions, including diagonally. Globe rupture is the only contraindication in evaluating the extraocular muscles.

Pupils

Note the size, shape, and reactivity of the pupils. A teardrop-shaped pupil often means a globe rupture. Some patients will have 1 to 2 mm of anisocoria (pupillary size difference); this can be normal. Afferent pupillary defect (APD) is determined by the swinging flashlight test. This test should be performed under slightly dim lighting conditions. Normally, both pupils will constrict when a light is shone into one eye. In normal eyes, swinging the light back and forth will keep both pupils constricted. If the eye has a process that blocks light to the optic nerve, that eye will dilate. Optic nerve dysfunction and large hemorrhages are two causes of an APD.

Sclera and Conjunctiva

The surface of the globe is composed of the conjunctiva, sclera, and cornea. The sclera is the white, tough collagenous part of the eye that anteriorly becomes the cornea. The conjunctiva is a thin vascular membrane that covers the sclera and inner eyelids.

Cornea

It is a thin, clear extension of the sclera. It is 500- to 600-μm thick, is very sensitive and is innervated by the fifth cranial nerve. See the fluorescein examination section for more on the cornea.

Anterior Chamber

This is the space between the iris and the cornea. It is filled with a clear fluid (the aqueous humor), which provides oxygen and nutrients to the cornea and lens. The slit lamp (see the following) is the best way to examine the anterior chamber.

SLIT LAMP

Patient Positioning

Have the patient sit facing the examiner, with his/her chin in the chinrest and forehead against the forehead strap (Figure 24.1). This will keep the patient's eyes within the focal range of the slit lamp.

Using the Slit Lamp

Although each slit lamp model is slightly different, the controls are generally similar (Figure 24.2). Most lamps use a joystick to focus. Elevation (getting the patient's eye in the center of your field) is first accomplished by grossly adjusting the chinrest up or down. The patient's eyes should be aligned with the black indicator marks on the slit lamp vertical bars. Fine tuning of elevation is then performed by spinning the joystick.

Once the eye is in focus, examine the lids/lashes for foreign bodies, debris, or lacerations. If a foreign body is suspected, be sure to evert (flip) the lids to examine behind each lid and deep into the corners.

To View the Anterior Chamber

Swing the light source on the slit lamp toward the temporal side of the patient's head and have it project at a sharp angle across the cornea. The area between the iris and cornea should be free of cells and debris. White blood cells floating in the anterior chamber are a result of inflammation. These often look like white dust

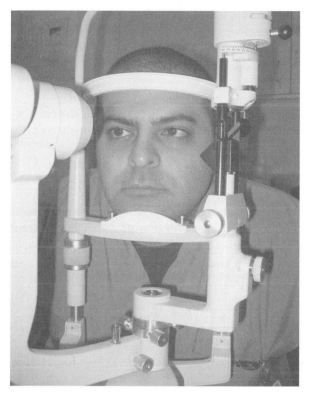

FIGURE 24.2 Slip lamp with person in proper position—note the chin resting.

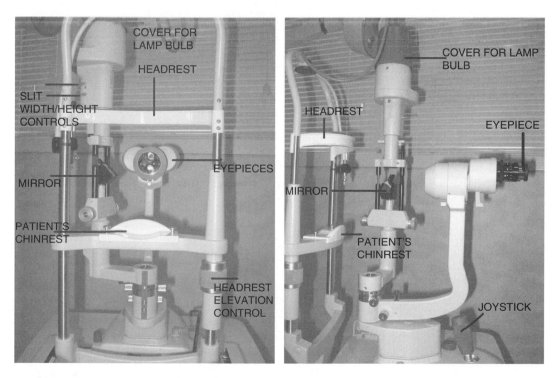

FIGURE 24.2 Slit lamp.

particles. "Flare" makes the anterior chamber look smoky and is a result of inflammatory proteins (note the term cells in flare). Here's where both hyphemas (blood) and hypopion (pus) are found.

Corneal Foreign Bodies and Abrasions

Shift the focus of the slit lamp to the superficial cornea. Frequently corneal foreign bodies can be seen without the use of fluorescein stain. Fluorescein is usually needed for the detection of abrasions.

To Use Fluorescein Stain

First instill a few drops of anesthetic (i.e., proparacaine or tetracaine). The easiest way to instill drops is to pull down the lower lid, creating a well. With the patient tilting his/her head back, drop several drops into the well created by the lid. Have the patient blink several times. Once the eye is anesthetized, drop 1 or 2 drops of the anesthetic onto the fluorescein strip, then touch the moistened strip to the same area where the anesthetic drops were placed—i.e., a well created by pulling down on the lower lid. Have the patient blink to distribute the stain.

Have the patient return to the slit lamp. Change the light source to cobalt blue. Again, focus on the superficial part of the cornea and look for any uptake. Corneal abrasions are usually linear; corneal ulcers are usually rounded and crater-like. Often with cloudy edges (edema), foreign bodies are also highlighted with the stain.

Multiple, linear, vertical abrasions suggest a foreign body under a lid. Be sure to examine under the lid.

INTRAOCULAR PRESSURE MEASUREMENT

Most emergency departments use an electronic intraocular pressure (IOP) measuring device, (i.e., Tono-Pen, Figure 24.3). The one contraindication to measuring the IOP is suspected globe rupture.

To Measure the IOP Using a Tono-Pen

Turn the device on. After confirming the device is calibrated, anesthetize the eye using drops. Place a cover (OCU-film) over the pen tip. With the patient supine,

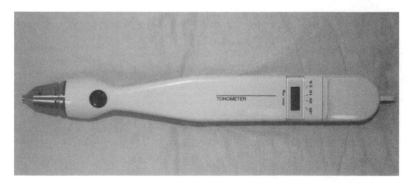

FIGURE 24.3
Commercial digital tonometer.

gently tap the tip onto the cornea several times; the average of three to four readings is used. The Tono-Pen will give the average of the readings with a bar under the statistical reliability of the readings. More than 20% is unreliable, and a repeat examination should proceed.

A reading below 20 mm Hg is normal; between 21 and 30 mm Hg should be referred for urgent ophthalmologic evaluation. Readings above 30 mm Hg require initiation of treatment to lower the IOP and emergent referral.

The Schiotz tonometer was historically used to measure IOP. However, other modalities such as the Tono-Pen and applanation tonometry have replaced this technique.

AUTHOR'S PEARLS

- *Be sure the tonometer is moving freely—test on the small plate that usually is attached to the box*
- *Be sure to rest your hand(s) while opening the lids on the orbital rim, not on the globe, as this will cause an increase in IOP*
- *Corneal ulcer cannot be missed and must be looked for*

RESOURCE

Varma, R. (1997). *Essentials of eye care: The Johns Hopkins Wilmer handbook* (pp. 26–38). Philadelphia: Lippincott Raven.

Managing Eye Injuries

LARRY ISAACS

FOREIGN BODY REMOVAL

Background

Although ocular trauma accounts for a small percentage of emergency department (ED) visits, its potential for life-changing consequences for the patient are high. During the initial assessment, there are questions to ask the patient that are important both for documentation and to provide clues to the nature of the injury. However, do not delay irrigation if indicated to ask these questions. The following is a partial list of questions to ask the patient: What was the patient doing? Does the patient wear contact lens or glasses? Was the patient wearing protective glasses? Is there a foreign body sensation? Was there a potential for a high-speed projectile?

Patient Presentation

- Pain
- Blurry vision
- Tearing
- Foreign body
- Body sensation

Treatment

First, one must determine if the foreign body is superficial or penetrating. Foreign body removal can be accomplished with a cotton-tipped applicator or needle, and/or irrigation. The suspected object and the location and depth of the object determine the type of removal. Prior to any assessment and intervention of the eye(s), a visual acuity should always be performed.

Contraindications and Relative Contraindications

- Open globe, intraocular foreign body

Special Considerations

- Some deep corneal foreign bodies may not be amenable to ED removal—referral to ophthalmology is appropriate
- A cooperative patient is necessary

Procedure Preparation

- Fluorescein stain
- Ophthalmic anesthetic (tetracaine)
- Cotton-tipped applicator
- Insulin syringe or small-gauge (27–30 gauge) needle with syringe
- Slit lamp
- Ophthalmoscope

Procedure

- Instill two drops of anesthetic
- With the patient in the slit lamp, use an insulin syringe and a cotton swab wetted with anesthetic
- Have the patient fix his/her gaze
- Rest your hand holding the syringe with your thumb and index fingers, resting your fifth digit and medial (ulnar) side of your hand on the patient's face (around the inferior orbital rim) for support
- While looking through the slit lamp, move the syringe slowly toward the patient's eye following the syringe needle as it comes into focus
- Once in focus with the bevel of the needle facing you, slowly and gently attempt to flick the foreign body out of the cornea (Figure 25.1)
- Do not dig deeply into the cornea
- Once out, it often sticks superficially to the cornea. Now, take the wetted cotton swab and touch it to the now-freed foreign body—it will often stick to the swab

RUST RING REMOVAL

Metallic foreign bodies will often leave a "rust ring"—a rust colored stain of the cornea. These patients will need follow-up with an ophthalmologist for removal of the rust ring. Topical antibiotics are indicated here, drops being more convenient for adults (i.e., polytrim) and ointment (erythromycin) for young children. If the patient wears contact lens, then the antibiotic choice should cover pseudomonas (i.e., ciprofloxacin, tobramycin, or gentamycin).

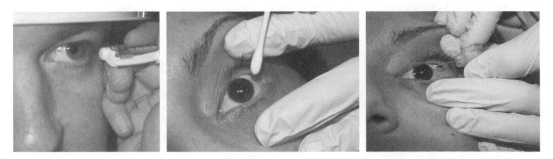

FIGURE 25.1 Foreign body removal from the eye.

Cyanoacrylate Glue

These glues can cause a chemical keratitis upon corneal contact. They also may attach to the lid margins. Do not force the lids open if glued shut. Applying petroleum-based products (erythromycin ointment, over-the-counter antibiotic ointment, or petroleum jelly) to the lids or placing on the cornea will degrade the glue in a short time.

Postprocedure Considerations

Rust rings should be addressed by an ophthalmologist. Cyanoacrylate glues on the cornea can leave a large, painful defect.

Educational Points

- Do not rub the eye
- Advise the patient that irritation may return when the anesthetic wears off but should resolve on its own
- Nonsteroidal anti-inflammatory medications can be taken for discomfort
- Antibiotic ointment is often prescribed
- Do not use an eye patch

Complications

- Corneal abrasion
- Infection

Author's Pearls

- *Don't cause more damage when attempting to remove a corneal foreign body; if it is deeply embedded, an ophthalmologist may be required*
- *Removal of a rust ring is not an emergency; here again, ophthalmology follow-up is all that is required*

CHEMICAL SUBSTANCE REMOVAL

Background

For both liquid and solid ocular injuries, the key is dilution with water. Even before a complete ocular examination, irrigation should begin. Use of either normal saline or lactated Ringer's is appropriate.

Patient Presentation

- Pain
- Burning
- Tearing
- Photophobia
- Blurry vision

Treatment

■ Immediate irrigation with normal saline or tap water if saline is not readily available.

Contraindications and Relative Contraindications

■ Open globe

Special Considerations

■ Alkaline versus acidic

Procedure Preparation

■ Ophthalmic anesthetic
■ Absorbent pads
■ Large basin
■ Normal saline or Ringer's lactate (liter bags intravenous [IV] solution)
■ IV tubing or commercial device (Morgan lens)
■ PH paper (litmus)

Procedure

INTRAVENOUS TUBING
■ Connect the normal saline or Ringer's lactate to the IV tubing and run it through
■ Instill several drops of anesthetic
■ Place an absorbent pad under the patient's head
■ Place the patient in Trendelenburg position
■ Place a large basin beneath the patient's head
■ Retract the eyelid
■ Instill several liters of fluid into the eye until a pH of 7.0 is achieved

MORGAN LENS
■ Retract the eyelids
■ Place an absorbent pad under the patient's head
■ Place the patient in Trendelenburg position
■ Place a large basin beneath the patient's head
■ Place the lens under both the upper and lower lid directly onto eye
■ Connect the normal saline or Ringer's lactate to the IV tubing and run it through
■ Instill several liters of fluid into the eye until a pH of 7.0 is achieved

Postprocedure Considerations

■ Check for corneal abrasions

Educational Points

■ Do not rub the eye
■ Advise the patient that irritation may return when the anesthetic wears off but should resolve on its own
■ Nonsteroidal anti-inflammatory medications can be taken for discomfort

> AUTHOR'S PEARL
>
> ■ *You can connect the end of the IV tubing to the end of a nasal cannula if irrigation of both eyes is required*

CONTACT LENS REMOVAL

Background

Most contact lens wearers can remove their own lenses. If they cannot find their lenses, you may need to assist with removal. Contact lenses may need to be removed for a full eye examination by the provider. Even lenses that are manufactured to be worn for long periods of time place the person at risk for *Pseudomonas* infection and corneal ulceration. Some contact lenses "fall out" of a person's eye without his or her knowledge. A full examination should be completed to ensure that the lens is not caught in the fornices.

Patient Presentation

■ Foreign body sensation
■ Pain
■ Redness
■ Irritation

Treatment

■ Removal of the contact lens is required

Procedure Preparation

■ Ophthalmic anesthetic drops
■ Fluorescein stain (may permanently discolor lens)
■ Cotton-tipped applicator
■ Normal saline and IV tubing
■ Commercially available suction cups

Procedure

First ask if they wear hard or soft lens. If the wearer cannot find the lens, it is usually up in the fornices (the deep corners behind the lids). Everting the lid may help find it.

■ You can use fluorescein, but remember that this will permanently discolor the lens
■ While placing traction on the lid, have the patient look to all four quadrants and often you will find the lens stuck to the globe
■ Sometimes anesthetic drops are necessary
■ A wet cotton-tipped applicator can also be used to move the lens
■ Once found, move it to the center of the cornea, where it can be removed
■ If the lens is adherent, irrigating with saline and a soft catheter will often loosen it
■ Soft contacts, once found, can be gently squeezed between the thumb and forefinger (this will break the suction)

- Irrigation will not break the seal when removing a hard lens. Commercially available suction cups will adhere to the lens for removal
- Always do a fluorescein examination after removal

Postprocedure Considerations

FLUORESCEIN STAIN UPTAKE
- If there is uptake, remember to prescribe an antipseudomonal antibiotic drop

Educational Points

- Do not wear contact lens until symptom free
- Follow-up with an optometrist/ophthalmologist

Complications

- Corneal abrasion

AUTHOR'S PEARL

- *Once you locate the lens, you can sometimes let the patient attempt removal.*

RESOURCES

Gifford, T. O., & Orlandi, R. R. (2008). Epistaxis. *Otolarngologic Clinics of North America, 41*(3), 525–536.
Kucik, C. J., & Clenney, T. (2005). Management of epistaxis. *American Family Physician, 71*(2), 305–312.

Procedures for Controlling Epistaxis

LARRY ISAACS

BACKGROUND

Epistaxis, or nose bleeding, is a common condition, usually self-limited, with a peak incidence from ages 2 to 10 and 50 to 80. Bleeding usually occurs when the mucosa erodes into superficial blood vessels. More than 90% of bleeding comes from the anterior area (Kiesselbach's plexus); posterior bleeds are harder to control, with increased risk of airway compromise and aspiration. With the exception of trauma, anterior epistaxis is most often unilateral. Posterior bleeding tends to be present in older patients and may cause bilateral epistaxis. The patient often complains of blood going down the back of the throat.

PATIENT PRESENTATION

- Bleeding from the nose and/or mouth
- Dizziness
- Skin—pale and sweaty
- Anxiety

TREATMENT

The treatment for epistaxis can be direct pressure, vasoconstrictors (phenylephrine), cautery (silver nitrate), or packing. Before any of these techniques, reassure the patient to alleviate anxiety; explain that identification of the source is imperative.

CONTRAINDICATIONS AND RELATIVE CONTRAINDICATIONS

- Significant facial fractures with suspected or confirmed basilar skull fracture

SPECIAL CONSIDERATIONS

Patients who are currently on antiplatelet agents (aspirin, NSAIDs, clopidogrel) or blood thinners, (i.e., warfarin, clopidogrel bisulfate, enoxaparin), and patients with uncontrolled hypertension are at greater risk for epistaxis. Treatment of underlying hypertension and coagulopathies will have an impact on the treatment.

PROCEDURE PREPARATION

- Personal protective equipment (gown, gloves, mask/eye shields)
- Absorbent pad
- Small or large basin
- Gauze
- Nose clip
- Cotton balls
- Vasoconstrictor
  - Oxymetazoline, phenylephrine, or 4% cocaine solution
- Lidocaine 4% or lidocaine 2% with epinephrine-soaked gauze
- Silver nitrate cautery
- Nasal packing/tampon
  - Ribbon gauze impregnated with petroleum jelly
  - Commercially prepared (Rhino Rocket, Gelfoam, Surgicel, and Floseal)
- Bayonet forceps

PROCEDURE

- Place absorbable pad on the upright patient's chest and have a basin on the lap
  - The basin is useful if patient spits up any blood or to place any used gauze and so on
- Have the patient blow the nose to remove any clots
- Have the patient hold direct, firm pressure on the external naris for 5 to 20 minutes, tilting the head forward (to prevent swallowing of blood)
- Instill a vasoconstrictor
  - Leave in for 10 to 15 minutes
  - This often temporarily stops the bleeding, giving you a view of the culprit vessel for definitive hemostasis
- Instill anesthesia
  - Lidocaine 4% or lidocaine 2% with epinephrine-soaked gauze
  - Leave in place for 5 to 10 minutes
- If the culprit vessel is seen, you can try to inject the area with a 27-gauge syringe using lidocaine 2% with epinephrine to achieve hemostasis

When hemostasis is achieved:

- The simplest way to achieve definitive treatment is by using silver nitrate cautery
- Locate the vessel/area of the bleeding
- Using one stick at a time, roll the tip on the mucosa until a dark gray eschar is formed
- Be sure to tell the patient that he or she may need to sneeze, so have the patient turn his or her head away from you and sneeze through the mouth

If silver nitrate is unable to achieve hemostasis, the site of bleeding is too difficult to locate, or the bleeding is too diffuse, the next step is some type of nasal packing/tampon:

- Layer the ribbon gauze from bottom to top
  - Layering the gauze (impregnated with petroleum jelly), from bottom to top does work, but it is time consuming

Commercial Product (Figure 26.1)

- Push the device with slow, gentle pressure into the naris on a horizontal plane, until the entire device is inside
- If the device has a balloon, have the patient tell you when he/she begins to feel the pressure as you inflate; that's when you stop
- Too much pressure can lead to pressure necrosis of the septum

Coat the dry packing devices with antibiotic ointment, rather than placing them dry. This helps with comfort and helps prevent toxic shock syndrome (having a tampon/packing in place puts the patient at risk for toxic shock).

- After the device is placed, examine the posterior pharynx
- Some blood behind the uvula is normal, and should stop; however, a constant flow of blood suggests a posterior bleed
- Posterior bleeds are more dangerous (because of aspiration risk and difficulty controlling the source)
- There are some commercial devices that control posterior bleeds (i.e., Rapid Rhino) but know that posterior bleeds should be admitted to the hospital

POSTPROCEDURE CONSIDERATIONS

- Antibiotic prophylaxis
- Antistaphylococcal coverage
  - Cephalexin or amoxicillin-clavulanate
  - Clindamycin or amoxicillin-clavulanate
- Referrel to an otolaryngologist for packing removal in 2 to 3 days

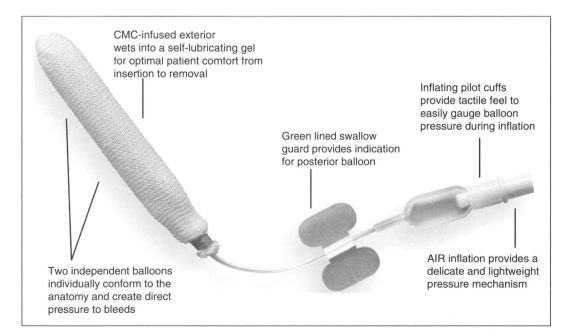

CMC-infused exterior wets into a self-lubricating gel for optimal patient comfort from insertion to removal

Green lined swallow guard provides indication for posterior balloon

Inflating pilot cuffs provide tactile feel to easily gauge balloon pressure during inflation

Two independent balloons individually conform to the anatomy and create direct pressure to bleeds

AIR inflation provides a delicate and lightweight pressure mechanism

FIGURE 26.1 Commercially available nasal tampon.

Source: Rapid Rhino image provided with permission from Arthrocare

EDUCATIONAL POINTS

- Do not remove the packing
- Do not blow the nose
- Sneeze with the mouth open
- Keep head elevated, avoid bending below the waist for 2 to 3 days

COMPLICATIONS

- Bleeding
- Toxic shock

Author's Pearls

- *Using ribbon gauze with bayonet forceps was, in the past, the standard way to pack a nose. Layering the gauze (impregnated with petroleum jelly), from bottom to top does work, but it is time consuming*
- *One of the many commercial devices (i.e., Rapid Rhino, Rhino Rocket, Gelfoam, Surgicel, Floseal) is certainly quicker and easier than ribbon gauze*
- *Follow the directions that come with the device (for the tampons). For products like Gelfoam/Surgicel, place a small piece of the product on the bleeding septum*

Procedure for Nasal Foreign Body Removal

LARRY ISAACS

BACKGROUND

This is usually a problem of young children, as adults rarely leave objects deep in their noses (except for psychiatric and mentally challenged adults). A history given by the parent or caregiver or a significant unilateral nasal discharge should prompt a search.

Nasal foreign bodies can be organic or nonorganic; they are commonly toys, beads, paper, nuts, and food. Button batteries can cause tissue erosion and ulceration, and if left in place for prolonged periods of time can lead to necrosis and septal perforation.

PATIENT PRESENTATION

- Pain
- Discharge
- Visible foreign body
- Anxiety

TREATMENT

Removal of the foreign body is necessary but not always achieved in the office, urgent, or emergency settings. In these cases, a referral to an otolaryngologist is required. Some foods, such as candy, usually dissolve before removal is possible.

SPECIAL CONSIDERATIONS

- Procedural sedation and sometimes the operating room/short procedure unit is required to remove deep objects

PROCEDURE PREPARATION

- Nasal speculum
- Good lighting
- Bayonet forceps or ear loop
- Vasoconstrictor
    - Oxymetazoline or phenylephrine
- Cyanoacrylate glue

- Cotton-tipped applicator (use the wooden end)
- 12-French foley catheter

PROCEDURE

- Using a nasal speculum is useful here and good lighting (either with an assistant holding a flashlight, good overhead lighting, or a headlamp)
- The proper way of holding the nasal speculum is to insert it into the naris with the handles horizontal (parallel to the floor)
- If you are able to visualize the object, using bayonet forceps or an earwax removal tool (with the tip bent at 90°) will often remove it
- If too much nasal discharge or bleeding, using a vasoconstrictor will help dry the naris of blood and/or mucous
- Topical anesthesia (lidocaine 4%) is helpful for patient comfort and cooperation

Parent Assisted Technique—"Parent's Kiss"

One technique that often works well is one that requires the parent's help. It works better with the larger objects (beans, large beads, and so on).

- Inform the parent that it may get a little "messy" when the object gets expelled. Having an absorbent pad on the patient's chest will help this somewhat
- With the patient being held by the parent (supine), have the parent occlude the unaffected naris and blow with a strong puff into the patient's mouth (Figure 27.1)
- This will often result in the object being expelled from the naris

Removal with 12-French Foley Catheter

- Apply vasocontrictor and topical anesthetic
- Slide the tip of the catheter into the naris beyond the object

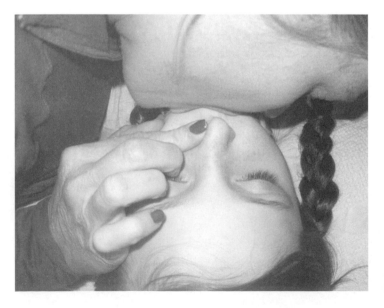

FIGURE 27.1 "Kiss" method of nasal foreign body removal.

- Slowly inflate the balloon with approximately 2 cc of air or water
- Slowly withdraw the catheter with the balloon inflated and remove the object

Cyanoacrylate Glue (Dermabond©, Indermil©)

- Be sure the naris is as dry as possible (using the vasoconstrictors)
- Place a drop of adhesive on the wooden tip of a cotton-tipped applicator
- Touch the foreign body with the wooden end and gently pull out of the naris

POSTPROCEDURE CONSIDERATIONS

- Try to be certain that all objects have been removed

EDUCATIONAL POINTS

- Unilateral foul-smelling nasal discharge in a young child/toddler is a nasal foreign body until proven otherwise

COMPLICATIONS

- There is sometimes epistaxis afterward—control as usual

AUTHOR'S PEARLS

- *Having the patient supine, in a parent's lap if necessary, is important. You will need some help holding the patient's head still. Note that sometimes procedural sedation may be necessary*
- *An alternative method to the "parent's kiss" is using a simple face mask over the mouth in which the provider blows the air while occluding the nare*

Procedure for Cerumen Removal

Theresa M. Campo

BACKGROUND

Cerumen, or ear wax, moisturizes as well as repels water in the auditory canal and is bacteriocidal and fungicidal. It is composed of lipids, complex proteins, and sugars. Cotton-tipped applicators that are used to clean the ears push the cerumen into the canal and pack it down, leading to obstruction. Patients usually don't present for treatment until they experience a "clogged" sensation, decreased or loss of hearing, fullness, and/or dizziness. Cerumen may partially or completely block the tympanic membrane and should be removed for a thorough examination.

Indications for this procedure include difficulty visualizing tympanic membrane, cerumen impaction, and debris removal associated with otitis externa.

PATIENT PRESENTATION

- Fullness in ear
- Blocked or clogged sensation
- Dizziness
- Loss of hearing
- Tinnitus
- Painless; if pain present, suspect other origin (i.e., infection or perforation)

TREATMENT

There are three methods of cerumen removal: curette, gentle suction, and warm water irrigation. Curette and irrigation are the most common and easily performed removals. Manual removal with curette is a simple procedure to perform for removing hard cerumen or large pieces. However, this can be painful to the patient. Warm water irrigation is painless, easy and more often used.

Ceruminolytic agents can also be used to soften and aid in the removal of cerumen. There are three types of ceruminolytic agents: water-based, oil-based, and non–water/non–oil based. These agents can be used alone or as pretreatment for curette or water irrigation removal.

CONTRAINDICATIONS AND RELATIVE CONTRAINDICATIONS

- History or suspicion for perforated tympanic membrane, severe canal swelling
- Previous pain with irrigation

- Previous surgery to middle ear
- History of middle ear disease
- Sharp or organic foreign bodies
- Tinnitus
- Vertigo
- Radiation therapy to external or middle ear, skull base or mastoid
- Patient with a history of mastoidectomy and hypersensitivity of the underlying structures

SPECIAL CONSIDERATIONS

- Patients who have previous surgery to the middle ear or mastoidectomy
- Diabetic patients should be carefully evaluated for the development of otitis externa after any manipulation of the ear and/or canal
- Irrigation should never be performed if a ruptured tympanic membrane is suspected or confirmed
- Jet irrigators can be used but care should be given not to rupture the tympanic membrane

PROCEDURE PREPARATION

Curette

- Flexible plastic or wire loop curette or plastic scoop
- Suction tip catheter or Frazier suction
- Gauze pads

Warm Water Irrigation

- Large volume syringe (30- to 60-mL) or ear irrigator tip and syringe
- Large gauge angiocatheter with needle removed (16 or 18 gauge)
- Warm water or normal saline
- Hydrogen peroxide
- Kidney basin
- Absorbent pad
- Towels

PROCEDURE

Curette

- Gently straighten the canal by pulling the pinna back and upward (downward for children)
- Visualize the canal and wax with the otoscope
- *Gently and slowly* insert the loop curette and remove the cerumen (Figure 28.1)

Warm Water Irrigation

- Place an absorbent pad over the patient's shoulder
- Have the patient sitting up with the kidney basin below the ear and held snug against the neck to prevent water running down onto the neck and shoulders
- Visualize the canal and wax with the otoscope

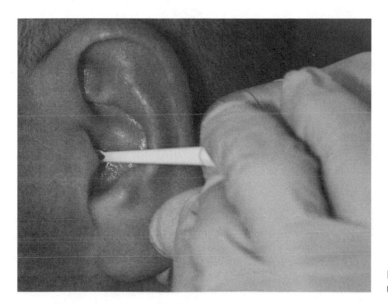

FIGURE 28.1 Cerumen removal with curette.

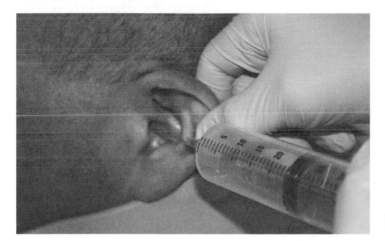

FIGURE 28.2 Cerumen removal with warm water irrigation.

- Fill the syringe with warm water
    - Use warm water to prevent discomfort and dizziness
    - Mix warm water and hydrogen peroxide (1:1 concentration)
- Gently straighten the canal by pulling the pinna back and upward (downward for children)
- Have the patient tilt his/her head so that the affected ear is facing the ground
- Instill the water gently and then allow it to run into the kidney basin (Figure 28.2)
- Repeat the irrigation until the cerumen is removed or the patient verbalizes complaints of pain, vertigo, and so on
- Use the curette to help remove cerumen that is pushed to the canal entrance
- Once completed, instill several drops of isopropanol in the canal to evaporate any residual moisture and prevent infection

POSTPROCEDURE CONSIDERATIONS

Pain

- The ear is very sensitive to pain
- Topical ear drops such as antipyrine and benzocaine can be given for pain relief

Tympanic Membrane

- Visualize the tympanic membrane to be sure it is intact and not perforated

Vertigo

- Have the patient lie down until the dizziness resolves, usually a few minutes
- If the vertigo persists, a short dosing period of antivertigo medications, such as meclizine, can be prescribed

Ear Canal Abrasion and/or Irritation

- Instillation and prescription of topical ear drops (i.e., fluoroquinolones) can be prescribed for the patient for a few days to help prevent infection and soothe the ear

EDUCATIONAL POINTS

- Do not use cotton-tipped applicators inside the ear canal
- Regular checkups with the primary care provider for evaluation and irrigation

COMPLICATIONS

- Diabetes and immunosuppression
  - Treat with a short regimen of topical antibiotic ear drops (i.e., fluoroquinolones) for a few days
- Complications arising from either curette or irrigation are usually benign and short lasting

---

AUTHOR'S PEARLS

- *Always try and have the patient assist in the removal by holding the basin and turning the head. It helps the patient feel as though he or she is helping with the removal*
- *Suction tip catheters can aid in the removal of the cerumen with either method. Use with caution in children*
- *Pretreatment with ceruminolytics can help with an easy and quick removal of cerumen*

RESOURCES

McCarter, D. F., Courtney, U., & Pollart, S. M. (2007). Cerumen impaction. *American Family Physician, 75*(10), 1523–1528, 1530.

O'Handley, J. G., Tobin, E., & Tagge, B. (2010). Otorhinolaryngology: Disorders of the external ear. In E. T. Bope, R. E. Rakel, & R. D. Kellerman (Eds.), *Conn's current therapy 2010* (1st ed.). Retrieved from http://www.mdconsult.com/das/book/body/188187220-3 /965596089/1481/281.html#4-u1.0-B978-1-4160-2467-5..50027-0–cesec69_1222

Riviello, R. J., & Brown, N. A. (2010). Otolaryngologic procedures. In J. R. Roberts & J. R. Hedges (Eds.), *Clinical procedures in emergency medicine* (5th ed., pp. 1189–1192). Philadelphia: Saunders Elsevier.

Procedure for Foreign Body Removal From the Ear Canal and Lobe

THERESA M. CAMPO

BACKGROUND

Foreign bodies in the external auditory canal are common complaints among children and adults. Foreign bodies can include insects, beads, rocks, sand, dirt, berries, vegetables, popcorn kernels, toys, cotton, erasers, and paper. The most common foreign body found in the ear is an insect. Removal of these foreign bodies is easier in the lateral canal than the medial canal because of sensory fibers.

Removal of foreign bodies can be distressing to the patient, especially a child. Limited attempts at removal should be made to help decrease anxiety and a painful, traumatic removal. Button batteries in the ear canal can cause significant tissue damage within hours, so immediate referral to an otolaryngologist should be done if prompt removal can't be completed. Foreign bodies located in the medial canal should also be referred to a specialist.

Occasionally, earring backs become embedded in the ear lobe. Inflammation from irritation or infection causes swelling of the lobe, which occurs around the earring back, especially if worn tightly. Removal by the patient is usually difficult because of anxiety and pain. Foreign body removal from the canal as well as the ear lobe will be discussed in this chapter.

PATIENT PRESENTATION

- Pain
  - Pain is severe if an insect is lodged in the canal
- Verbalization to the parent or other person by a child
- Fullness
- Vertigo
- Feel and hear something "moving" or "buzzing"

TREATMENT

There are numerous methods for removal of foreign bodies. The type of method used may depend upon the particular object you are attempting to remove. Irrigation, as discussed in Chapter 28, is most helpful for removal of dirt, sand, or small objects lying near the tympanic membrane. Irrigation should not be used for removal of organic material such as vegetables, seeds, and so on, because the water causes the object to swell, making removal more difficult. Suction tip catheters can be used for removal of difficult-to-grab objects such as beads and other smooth, round objects. These round objects become lodged in the canal because of the oval shape of the ear canal. Manual removal with various types of curettes can be used to remove small objects, where the curette can be passed along the side of the object and gently pulled out of the canal. This method can be uncomfortable because of the sensitivity and nerve innervations of the canal. Alligator forceps can be used to remove objects that are easily grabbed, for example, insects, paper, cotton, and so on. Glue (cyanoacrylate) can also be used for removal of dry, smooth, and round objects in the lateral canal.

CONTRAINDICATIONS AND RELATIVE CONTRAINDICATIONS

- Irrigation should not be performed if suspicion or confirmation of tympanic membrane rupture or perforation are present

SPECIAL CONSIDERATIONS

- Patients who are extremely anxious
  - Consider conscious sedation or referral to an otolaryngologist for these patients to avoid traumatic removal

PROCEDURE PREPARATION

All Procedures

- Gloves
- Gauze pads
- Absorbent pads

Suction Tip Catheter

- Suction tip catheter (Frazier suction)

Manual Removal

- Flexible or rigid curette (loop or scoop)
- Alligator forceps

Insect Removal

- Mineral oil
- Lidocaine solution (2% or 4%)
- Alligator forceps and/or curette

Glue (Cyanoacrylate)

- Paper clip, cotton-tipped applicator, very thin paint brush
- Glue

PROCEDURE

Suction Tip Catheter

- Inform the patient of the suction catheter noise so he or she is prepared and not startled
  - Allowing the patient to hear the suction beforehand can alleviate fear
- Place the suction between 100 and 140 mm Hg
- Gently straighten the canal by pulling the pinna back and upward for adults or downward for children
- Gently place the suction tip onto the object and begin to suction and pull the object out of the canal (Figure 29.1)
  - Keep the tip away from the canal wall

Manual Removal

- Gently straighten the canal by pulling the pinna back and upward for adults or downward for children
- Visualize the canal and foreign body with the otoscope
- *Gently and slowly* insert the loop curette and remove the foreign body (Figure 29.2)

Insect Removal

- Instill either mineral oil and/or lidocaine (2% or 4%)
  - Mineral oil has been shown to be more effective
- Once the insect is dead, removal with mechanical technique can be performed

Glue (Cyanoacrylate)

- Place a small amount of glue on the tip of either a straightened paper clip, blunt/wooden end of a cotton-tipped applicator, or a very thin paintbrush

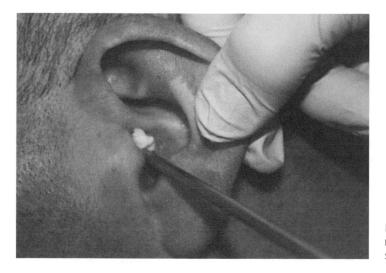

FIGURE 29.1 Foreign body removal from the ear with a suction tip catheter.

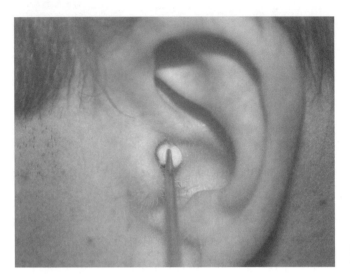

FIGURE 29.2 Manual removal of a foreign body from the ear.

- Once the glue is tacky straighten the canal, as described earlier, and place the tip against the object and gently pull out of the canal

This procedure is best used in cooperative adults. Glue can possibly spill or drip into the canal or the end of the applicator can adhere to the canal. Precision and patience is key with this procedure.

Earring Back in Earlobe

- Wipe the area clean with gauze and normal saline
- Grasp the earlobe with both thumbs and index fingers
- Gently, but firmly, push the anterior side toward the posterior side allowing the earring back to rise between your thumbs
- Remove the back from the earring post
- Remove the entire earring
- Irrigate with normal saline
- Apply topical antibiotic if necessary
- Patients should not replace earring until healed

POSTPROCEDURE CONSIDERATIONS

- Minor abrasions usually heal without complications
- Topical antibiotic drops can be prescribed to help prevent infection but have not been proven to be effective or necessary

EDUCATIONAL POINTS

- Children
  - Do not put anything in the ears, nose, or other "holes" in their bodies
  - Do not put anything smaller than your elbow in the ear

- Adults
  - Do not use cotton-tipped applicators
- Insects
  - Pest control should be advised in those patients with insects that occur while sleeping or in the home
  - Some insects just "fly in" especially during the warmer months

COMPLICATIONS

- Tympanic rupture/perforation can occur either from the foreign body or from a traumatic removal

---

AUTHOR'S PEARLS

- *If a patient presents with a chronic dry cough that is not resolving, check the external canal for foreign body. It may be pressing on the tenth cranial nerve causing the cough*
- *Always evaluate the other ear and nose for additional foreign bodies in children*
- *Always perform and document your evaluation before and after removal, including removal failure*
- *Cooperation and immobilization are key to a successful foreign body removal*

RESOURCES

Heim, S. W., & Maughan, K. L. (2007). Foreign bodies in the ear, nose, and throat. *American Family Physician, 76*(8), 1185–1189.

Mantooth, R. (2009). Foreign bodies, ear. Retrieved from http://emedicine.com/article/763712-overview and http://emedicine.com/article/763712-treatment

O'Handley, J. G., Tobin, E., & Tagge, B. (2010). Otorhinolaryngology: Disorders of the external ear. In E. T. Bope, R. E. Rakel, & R. D. Kellerman (Eds.), *Conn's current therapy 2010* (1st ed.). Retrieved from http://www.mdconsult.com/das/book/body/188187220-3/965596089/1481/281.html#4-u1.0-B978-1-4160-2467-5..50027-0–cesec69_1222

Riviello, R. J., & Brown, N. A. (2010). Otolaryngologic procedures. In J. R. Roberts & J. R. Hedges (Eds.), *Clinical procedures in emergency medicine* (5th ed., pp. 1194–1195). Philadelphia: Saunders Elsevier.

Procedure for Managing an Auricular Hematoma

THERESA M. CAMPO

BACKGROUND

An auricular hematoma occurs from direct, blunt trauma to the ear causing a shearing force. It is commonly seen in wrestlers, rugby players, and after an assault or altercation. The shearing of the anterior auricle leads to separation of the perichondrium and the underlying vessels, leading to hematoma formation and compromise to the avascular cartilage. This injury needs immediate treatment to prevent the development of cauliflower ear and infection. Cauliflower ear is the development of new chaotic cartilage formation, which leads to a chronic and permanently deformed ear.

PATIENT PRESENTATION

■ Anterior auricular tenderness, swelling, and/or deformity following trauma

TREATMENT

Treatment should be immediate to prevent complications. Needle aspiration and incision and drainage are the treatments of choice. Consideration should be given to needle aspiration as recurrence and difficulties producing full evacuation are considerable concerns. Treatment goals are to completely drain and evacuate the hematoma and prevent reaccumulation of the hematoma with a pressure dressing. Needle aspiration and incision and drainage techniques will be discussed in this chapter.

Regardless of technique, patients should be placed on antistaphylococcal antibiotics and close follow-up should be discussed with the patient and family members.

CONTRAINDICATIONS AND RELATIVE CONTRAINDICATIONS

■ Hematoma more than 7 to 10 days old
■ Recurrent or chronic hematoma

SPECIAL CONSIDERATIONS

■ Pediatric patient
  ■ Conscious sedation may be necessary for deep-seated or difficult-to-manage areas because of movement or severity
  ■ Each case should be considered independently

■ Immunocompromised or have comorbidities
  ■ Patients with organ transplant, HIV-AIDS, diabetes, and/or cancer
■ Pregnancy
  ■ Antibiotics that are considered to be safe in pregnancy should be prescribed if necessary

PROCEDURE PREPARATION

Needle Aspiration

■ 18- to 20-gauge needle
■ 10-mL syringe
■ Topical antibiotic ointment

Incision and Drainage

■ 3-mL syringe with 23- to 27-gauge needle—anesthesia
■ Lidocaine 1% *without* epinephrine—anesthesia
■ No. 11 or No. 15 blade scalpel
■ 20-mL syringe with 18-gauge angiocatheter and normal saline for irrigation
■ Topical antibiotic ointment

Compression Dressing

■ 4 × 4 Gauze
■ Stretch bandage/roll gauze
■ Dry cotton
■ Vaseline gauze, 1/4 inch, plain packing, or saline-soaked gauze

Sutured Dental Rolls

■ Dental rolls
■ 4-0 Nylon suture material
■ Suture kit

PROCEDURE

Small Hematoma

NEEDLE ASPIRATION
■ Prepare the site with skin cleanser and dry with a 4 × 4 gauze
■ Attach the 18- to 20-gauge needle to the 10-mL syringe
■ Insert the needle into the hematoma (Figure 30.1)
■ "Milk" the hematoma between your thumb and forefinger until the contents are completely drained
■ Withdraw the needle from the ear
■ Apply a simple compression dressing to the ear to prevent reaccumulation (see the following)

INCISION AND DRAINAGE
■ Place the patient in the lateral decubitus position with the affected ear facing upward

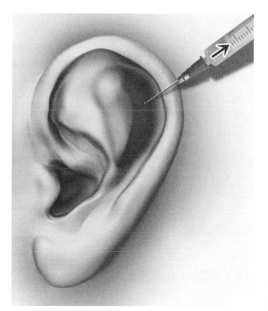

FIGURE 30.1 Needle aspiration of an auricular hematoma.

- Prepare the area with skin cleanser
- Dry the area with a 4 × 4 gauze
- Perform local infiltration with the lidocaine 1% *without* epinephrine (an auricular block can also be performed; see Chapter 9)
- Using the scalpel, incise along the natural skin fold of the anterior auricle following the curve of the pinna (Figure 30.2)
- Gently peel the skin and perichondrium off the hematoma
- Completely evacuate the hematoma (suction may be used if necessary)
- Draw the saline into the large syringe
- Apply the splash shield to the end of the syringe
- Irrigate the area
- Dry thoroughly
- Apply topical antibiotic ointment and approximate the wound edges
- Apply a pressure dressing or suture dental rolls to the ear; both are described in the following sections

COMPRESSION DRESSING
- Insert dry cotton into ear canal
- Mold the conforming gauze into the convolutions of the ear (Vaseline, saline, or packing)
- Cut a "V" shape into the 4 × 4 gauze to allow for a snug and comfortable fit behind the ear and place behind the entire ear
- Place multiple layers of gauze over the ear
- Wrap stretch bandage/roll gauze around the head to secure the dressing in place (Figure 30.3)

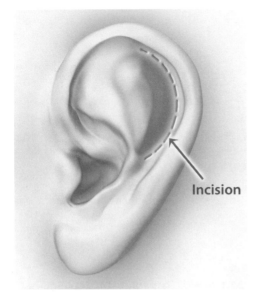

FIGURE 30.2 Incision and drainage of an auricular hematoma.

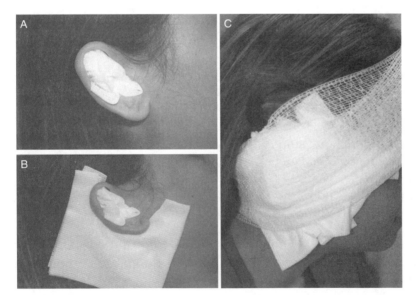

FIGURE 30.3
Application of compression dressing.

SUTURED DENTAL ROLLS
- With 4-0 nylon suture material, pass over the hematoma through the entire thickness of the ear
- Place the dental roll on the posterior aspect of the ear and wrap the suture material over it
- Pass the suture needle back through the pinna such that it comes out anteriorly

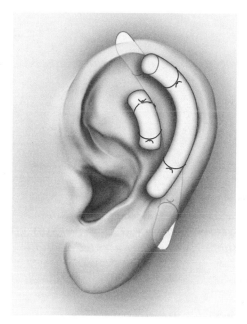

FIGURE 30.4 Suture dental rolls.

- Place another dental roll on the anterior aspect of the pinna over the incision
- Wrap the suture material over the dental roll and tie into place (Figure 30.4)
- Remove dressing in 7 days

POSTPROCEDURE CONSIDERATIONS

Recurrence

Drainage may need to be repeated if fluid reaccumulation occurs

- Referral to specialist is indicated

EDUCATIONAL POINTS

- Close follow-up every 24 hours is necessary to assess for recurrence, infection, and vascular compromise
- Aspirin, nonsteroidal anti-inflammatory medication, or anticoagulant medications should be avoided to prevent recurrence

COMPLICATIONS

- Reaccumulation of the hematoma is the most common complication seen
- Infection, chondritis, and scar formation
- Early drainage and close monitoring can help prevent the development of scar tissue (cauliflower ear). However, it may still develop
- Recurrence and infection are indications for surgical treatment and intravenous antibiotics

AUTHOR'S PEARLS

■ *Discuss with the patient the possibility of reoccurrence and development of cauliflower ear*

■ *Premedicate with oral analgesia medication*

■ *Reassurance should be given to patients of any age*

■ *Drainage should be performed on all hematomas unless it is older than 7 days*

■ *The use of lidocaine with epinephrine has generally been contraindicated for the outer ear. However, recent literature suggests that the use of epinephrine does not block the circulation to this area of the ear and, therefore, does not cause necrosis. The decision to use epinephrine for local infiltration of the outer ear is at the clinician's discretion and should be based on the most up-to-date evidence practice. Epinephrine is also acceptable for regional block of the ear*

RESOURCES

Leybell, I. (2009). Drainage, auricular hematoma. Retrieved from http://emedicine.com/article/82793-overview and http://emedicine.com/article/82793-treatment

O'Handley, J. G., Tobin, E., & Tagge, B. (2010). Otorhinolaryngology: Disorders of the external ear. In E. T. Bope, R. E. Rakel & R. D. Kellerman (Eds.), *Conn's current therapy 2010* (1st ed.). Retrieved from http://www.mdconsult.com/das/book/body/188187220-3/965596089/1481/281.html#4-u1.0-B978-1-4160-2467-5..50027-0–cesec69_1222

Riviello, R. J., & Brown, N. A. (2010). Otolaryngologic procedures. In J. R. Roberts & J. R. Hedges (Eds.), *Clinical procedures in emergency medicine* (5th ed., pp. 1195–1197). Philadelphia: Saunders Elsevier.

31

Dental Anatomy, Examination, and Anesthetics

Theresa M. Campo

DENTAL ANATOMY

The tooth is composed of the crown and root. The crown is the visible part and is covered with enamel. It projects above the gingiva and consists of three layers. The outer layer is the enamel and is the hardest structure of the tooth with increased mineralization. The center layer is the dentin, a bone-like material, and the pulp is the inner hollow layer.

The root system is also composed of three layers: the cementum (outer layer), dentin (middle layer), and the pulp canal (the center). Blood vessels and nerves enter the pulp through the apical foramen and pulp canal. The pulp supplies the dentin with nutrients. Periodontal ligaments act as a sling or hammock holding the tooth in the socket and cushioning the tooth during mastication. These ligaments secure the tooth to the alveolar bone (Figure 31.1).

There are primary and secondary teeth. Primary teeth, also known as milk or baby teeth, consist of 20 teeth that begin to erupt at around 6 months of age and are complete at about 2 years of age. These teeth begin to shed between age 6 and 12 years and are complete around the 18th birthday. Secondary teeth, or permanent teeth, consist of 32 teeth: 8 incisors, 4 canine, 8 premolars, and 12 molars.

The teeth can be divided into two areas: the upper and lower arches (maxillary and mandibular teeth). These areas can be further divided into the four areas of upper and lower, right and left. They are referenced to the patient (i.e., patient's right upper or left lower). There are four groups of teeth: the incisors, canines, premolars, and molars.

The incisors are the four most anterior maxillary and mandibular teeth and are responsible for cutting and biting food. They have one root. There are four canine teeth (maxillary and mandibular), which are just distal to the incisors. They are responsible for ripping and tearing food and are the longest and most stable of the teeth. They have one root.

The next teeth are the premolars with four each in the maxilla and mandible. They have sharp points and a broad base for ripping, chewing, and grinding food. The premolars have one root but the first maxillary may have two roots. The molars are the farthest back, a with six each in the maxilla and mandible. They consist of a broad surface for crushing, chewing, and grinding food. They may have one to four roots. The third molars maxillary and mandibular are called wisdom teeth.

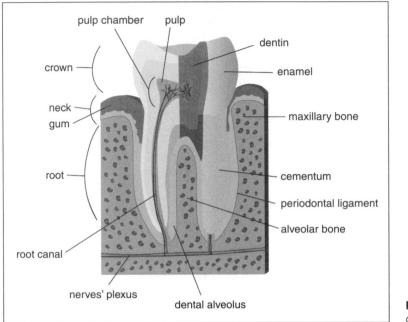

FIGURE 31.1 Tooth anatomy.

DENTAL EXAMINATION

A thorough examination of the oral cavity should be done with any complaints of facial swelling, sore throat, sinus pressure, neck, or oral pain, swelling, or drainage. Before starting an examination the patient should be asked to remove any dentures or removable appliances for full visualization.

INSPECTION

- External features of the face and neck
- Jaw movement for symmetry
- Lips

INTRA ORAL

- Mucosa and tissue including frenula
  - Torn frenulum can be a sign of abuse

GINGIVA

- Inflammation could be a sign of systemic disease (i.e., diabetes or pregnancy)

TEETH

- There are 32 permanent teeth. Numbering begins with the right upper molar (No. 1) counting across to the left upper molar (No. 16) followed by the left lower molar (No. 17) and finishing at the right lower molar (No. 32) (Figure 31.2)
- Discoloration can be from medications or poor hygiene

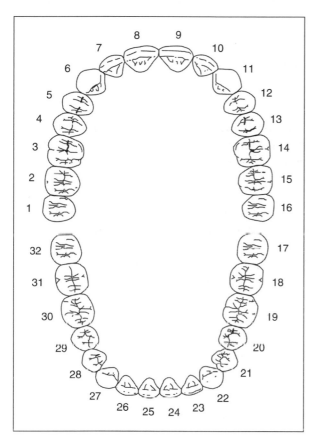

FIGURE 31.2 Numbering of teeth.

TONGUE

■ Lesions, cuts, or bleeding

HARD AND SOFT PALATE

■ Lesions
■ Have patient say "Ahhh" and note symmetrical rise of uvula/palate

PALPATION

■ Periauricular, submandibular, submental, and cervical lymph nodes
■ Temporalmandibular joint
   ■ Symmetry of movement
   ■ Clicking or crepitus
■ Intraoral tissue including the frenula
■ Gingiva
■ Teeth
   ■ Chipping, break, roughness, and mobility
■ Express Wharton's duct
   ■ Located under tongue
   ■ Fluid should be clear

■ Hard and soft palate
  ■ Masses

ANESTHETICS

Background

Dental anesthesia is used for many dental, oral, and maxillofacial procedures including odontalgia (toothache) and lacerations. Dental blocks do not distort soft tissue needing repair and is a safe way to control pain without the use of narcotics.

Profound anesthesia can be achieved through infiltration or depositing anesthetic apically to a particular tooth. This can be accomplished for all teeth in the mouth with the exception of the lower molars. The lower molars usually require a mandibular block (inferior alveolar infiltration/lingual infiltration). Infiltration typically provides profound anesthesia to the tooth after approximately 7 minutes. The mandibular block can take up to 15 minutes to achieve profound anesthesia.

Treatment

Dental anesthesia can be helpful with the following:

■ Odontalgia and pulpitis
■ Dental impaction
■ Periodontal abscess
■ Laceration repair of the tongue, lip, and oral mucosa
■ Dental, mandibular, and/or maxillary fractures and trauma

Contraindications and Relative Contraindications

■ Hypersensitivity or allergies to anesthetic agents
■ Uncooperative patients
■ Infected tissue
■ Bleeding disorders
■ Valvular heart disease

Special Considerations

■ Proper documentation of a patient with a history of neurovascular damage.

Procedure Preparation

■ Lidocaine 5% or benzocaine 20% solution for topical application
■ Nonsterile gloves
■ Absorbent pads
■ Gauze
■ Cotton-tipped applicator(s) or cotton balls
■ Lidocaine 1% or 2% or bupivacaine 0.25% with or without epinephrine
■ 3-mL syringe
■ Small gauge needle (25- to 27-gauge)
■ Suction set-up with Yankauer suction tip

Procedure

TOPICAL

Topical anesthesia can be beneficial to reduce the pain experienced with injectable anesthesia.

- Dry mucosa with gauze
- Place lidocaine 5% or benzocaine 20% solution on the tip of applicators or cotton balls
- Place on mucosa where needle is to be inserted for 3 to 5 minutes (Figure 31.3)

INJECTABLE

Injectable anesthesia can be used for laceration repair, mandibular fractures, toothache, and abscess. Lidocaine 1% or 2% with or without epinephrine can be used for lacerations (short term) or bupivacaine 0.25% with or without epinephrine can be used for mandibular fractures or toothaches (long term) for their respective durations.

SUPRAPERIOSTEAL INFILTRATION (LOCAL)
Individual tooth pain or toothache:

- Apply topical anesthetic described previously
- Have the patient relax their facial muscles as much as possible by asking to close his/her mouth
- Fully extend the mucous membrane for visualization by either pulling gently out and down (mandibular) or out and up (maxilla)
- Dry the area with gauze and visualize the mucobuccal fold
- Insert the needle into the mucous fold, in front of the affected tooth, with the bevel of the needle facing the bone (Figure 31.4)
- Aspirate
- Inject 1 to 2 mL of anesthetic at the apex of the tooth
- Withdraw the needle
- Give patient gauze to hold pressure
- If the procedure fails to anesthetize the area, inject the palatal side of the tooth. This procedure may not be as effective on back molars.

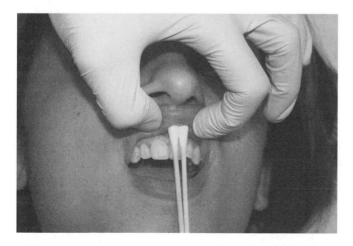

FIGURE 31.3 Topical anesthetic.

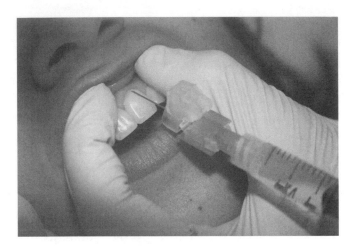

FIGURE 31.4 Supraperiosteal infiltration.

ANTERIOR SUPERIOR ALVEOLAR BLOCK
Canine and incisors (lateral and medial):

- Apply topical anesthetic
- Have the patient relax the upper lip by closing the jaw slightly
- Retract the lip anteriorly
- Insert the needle at the apex of the canine tooth at a 45° angle (Figure 31.5)
- Aspirate
- Inject 2 mL of anesthetic
- Withdraw the needle
- Give patient gauze to hold pressure

MIDDLE SUPERIOR ALVEOLAR BLOCK (MSA)
Mediobuccal root of maxillary first molar:

- Apply topical anesthetic
- Have the patient open his/her mouth about half way
- Retract the cheek laterally
- Position and insert the needle at the junction between the second premolar and first molar at a 45° angle (Figure 31.6)
- Aspirate
- Inject 2 to 3 mL of anesthetic
- Withdraw the needle
- Give patient gauze to hold pressure

POSTERIOR OR SUPERIOR ALVEOLAR BLOCK
Maxillary molars:

- Apply topical anesthetic
- Have the patient open the mouth about half way
- Retract the cheek laterally
- Position the needle to the posterior aspect of the second molar and insert toward the maxillary tuberosity (upward, backward, and inward) along the curvature of the tuberosity approximately 2 to 2.5 cm (Figure 31.7)

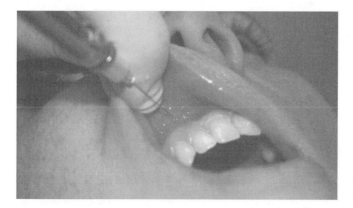

FIGURE 31.5 Anterior superior alveolar block.

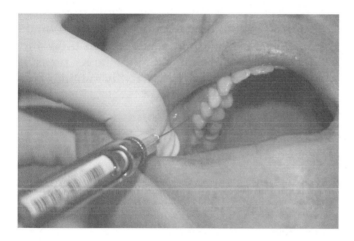

FIGURE 31.6 Middle superior alveolar block.

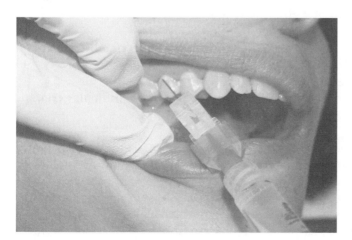

FIGURE 31.7 Posterior superior alveolar block.

- Aspirate
- Inject 2 to 3 mL of anesthetic
- Withdraw the needle
- Give patient gauze to hold pressure
- Occasionally the first molar will not be anesthetized with this technique alone and will need an additional technique (MSA)
- Puncture of the pterygoid plexus and hematoma formation can occur if aspiration is not performedw
- Cranial nerve V can be blocked if the needle is inserted too far posteriorly

Upper molars and upper first premolars may require a palatal injection due to these teeth possessing a palatal root. Determine about where the root tip would be in the palate and press a blunt object with gentle pressure (such as the blunt end of the dental mirror). At the same time, insert the needle into the tissue near the mirror handle. Slowly express a small amount of anesthetic into the site. Only use a small amount (few drops), and tissue blanching is a good indication of enough anesthetic. Too much anesthetic with the pressure applied can result in necrosis. This procedure is well tolerated due to the Gate theory of pain, which states that the larger pressure nerve fibers will override the smaller pain nerve fibers. This is why rubbing your head after you hit it is soothing.

Inferior Alveolar Infiltration (With Lingual Nerve Block)

Most common type of dental nerve block used to anesthetize the mandibular teeth to midline, floor of the mouth, lower lip, chin, and anterior two-third of tongue. Although this technique may be considered more complex than previous methods, once mastered it is a highly effective block. It should be performed after viewing material and with supervision until proficient in this technique.

- Have the patient lying down with the back of the head firmly against the stretcher or in a reclining position in a dental chair, if available
- Stand on the side opposite of the area to be injected
- Palpate the coronoid notch and then place the thumb over the notch (retromolar fossa—anterior ramus of the mandible)
- Place the index finger just anterior to the ear (external ramus)
- Retract the tissue toward the cheek and visualize the pterygomandicular triangle (see Figure 31.8)
- Apply topical anesthetic
- Hold the syringe parallel to the mandibular teeth at an angle to the medial ramus with the distal end of the syringe lying between the first and second premolars on the opposite side of the mouth
- In children, the syringe will need to be held at a slightly higher angle not parallel because of the difference in anatomy (mandibular foramen is lower)
- Insert the needle into the triangle approximately 1 cm above the level of the teeth until the end of the needle hits the bone (usually no more than 2.5 cm)
- Withdraw the needle slightly, aspirate, and then instill the anesthetic
    - 5 mL

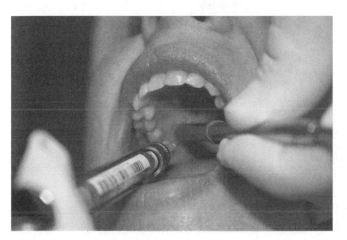

FIGURE 31.8 Inferior block.

- The lingual nerve can also be anesthetized as it branches off of the inferior alveolar nerve at this point

Patients may experience jaw soreness after the injection for a few days. Be sure to include this information in your instructions.

Mental Nerve Infiltration

This block is most commonly used for lower lip lacerations. The mental nerve is an extension of the inferior alveolar nerve through the mental foramen. This nerve block can be performed either intraoral or extraoral. However, the intraoral technique will only be covered in this book as it is considered to be less painful to the patient.

- Palpate the mental foramen by placing a gloved finger over the labial fold over the mandible approximately 1 cm inferior and anterior to the second premolar
  - Between the first and second premolar in adults
  - Between the first and second primary molars in children
- Apply topical anesthetic
- Insert the needle at a 45° angle using the supraperiosteal technique
  - Do not inject directly into the foramen as this can cause nerve damage
- Aspirate and then instill 2 to 3 mL of anesthetic while "fanning out" (see Figure 31.9).

Educational Points

- Warm salt water rinses
- Caution with chewing and swallowing food due to anesthesia
- Caution with swallowing of fluids due to anesthesia

Complications

- Pain
- Infection
- Allergic reaction
- Anxiety

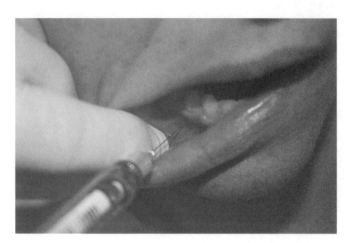

FIGURE 31.9 Mental block.

AUTHOR'S PEARLS

- *Distraction through imagery can help to decrease the patients anxiety*
- *Having the parent at the bedside for comfort*
- *Massaging the injection site can help increase the speed of absorption*
- *Make sure the periosteum is encountered when performing inferior nerve anesthesia*
- *Recent literature shows a link between periodontal and myocardial infarctions as the increased inflammatory activity in atherosclerotic lesions may represent a link between periodontal infection and cardiovascular disease*
- *An apprehensive patient or pulp infection may require additional anesthetic*

RESOURCES

Bahekar, A. A., Singh, S., Saha, S., Molnar, J., & Arora, R. (2007). The prevalence and incidence of coronary heart disease is significantly increased in periodontitis: A meta-analysis. *American Heart Journal 154*(5), DOI: 10.1016/j.ahj.2007.06.037.

Benko, R. (2010). Regional anesthesia of the head and neck. In J. R. Roberts & J. R. Hedges (Eds.), *Clinical procedures in emergency medicine* (5th ed., pp. 1217–1219, & 503–506). Philadelphia: Saunders Elsevier.

Hermann, H. J., & Laskin, D. M. (2007). In P. S. Auerbach (Ed.), *Wilderness medicine* (5th ed.). Philadelphia: Mosby Elsevier. Retrieved from http://www.mdconsult.com/das/book/body/188210824–3/0/1483/238.html?tocnode=54235634&fromURL=238.html#4-u1.0-B978–0-323–03228-5..50031–8_1433

Knight, J. (2009). Dental basics for primary care NPs. *The American Journal for Nurse Practitioners, 13*(3), 36–41.

Scheinfeld, N. S. (2009, May 17) Nerve block, inferior alveolar. Retrieved from http://emedicine.medscape.com/article/82622-overview and http://emedicine.medscape.com/article/82622-treatment

Van Meter, M. W., & Dave, A. K. (2009, April 5). Nerve block, oral. Retrieved from http://emedicine.medscape.com/article/82850-overview & http://emedicine.medscape.com/article/82850-treatment

32

Procedures for Managing Dental Injuries

Theresa M. Campo

INTRODUCTION

Dental pain and injuries are commonly seen in the emergency and urgent care settings and less frequently in the office setting. They can be anxiety producing for the patient and family members. Dentoalveolar abscesses, odontalgia (toothache), dental fractures, and luxations are the most common problems requiring quick interventions. Other problems encountered by providers are pulpitis, gingivitis, pericoronitis, cellulitis, and periodontitis, which will not be covered in this chapter.

In the United States in 2008, dental services accounted for $101.2 billion of the $2.3 trillion spent on health care. Direct costs accompanied by the indirect costs of days lost at school and work are not only a burden financially on the individual and family but also on society. Providers can address these problems early and efficiently through procedures, medical treatment, and referral to dentists and oral surgeons.

DENTOALVEOLAR ABSCESS

Background

Dentoalveolar abscesses are a collection of pus in the structures surrounding the teeth. In children, the abscess is usually periapical from dental caries invading the protective layer and the pulp. The infection causes pulpitis (inflammation of the pulp) and may lead to necrosis. The abscess is formed when the infection reaches the alveolar bone. A periodontal abscess is more common in adults and involves the periodontal ligaments and bone (support structures). This type of abscess can occur secondary to foreign body in children. Infections are polymicrobial with anaerobic gram-negative rods and gram-positive cocci, facultative and microaerophilic streptococci, and viridans streptococci.

Deep space infections present with fever, trismus, toxic appearance, chills, pain, and difficulty with speech and/or swallowing. The infection can spread into the deep spaces of the face and neck. These spaces include buccal, maxillary sinus, parapharyngeal, retropharyngeal, sublingual, submandibular, submasseteric, temporal, and others. The sublingual space can cause elevation of the base of the tongue and floor of the mouth, causing dysphagia and airway compromise.

Patient Presentation

- Pain (buccal and/or facial; local or along facial planes)
- Swelling (intraoral and/or extraoral)
  - Common locations and associated cause of facial swelling are given in Table 32.1
- Fever
- Gingival bleeding
- Pus drainage
- Regional lymphadenopathy (submental, submandibular, cervical)
- Fluctuant mass (buccal or palatal)

TABLE 32.1 Facial Swelling

Region	Location/Cause	Presentation

*Sublingual	Mandibular
	Canine
	Lateral and medial
	  incisors
	Premolar
	First molar
		Pain
		Dysphagia
		Unilateral elevation floor
		  of mouth and/or base of
		  tongue
		Airway compromise

*Submandibular	Mandibular
	Second molar
	Third molar
		Pain
		Swelling—triangle of neck
		  around angle of jaw (below
		  mandible)
		Trismus
		Tender to palpation

*Submental	Mandibular
	  incisors
		Pain
		Firm
		Midline swelling beneath
		  chin

Retropharyngeal (more common in children of 4 years and younger)	Maxillary or mandibular First molar Second molar Third molar	Stiff neck Sore throat Dysphagia Voice change Stridor (sever case involving mediastinum)
Buccal	Maxillary or mandibular Premolar Molar	Pain Swollen cheeks Trismus

Masticator	Mandibular
	Third molar
		Pain
		Trismus
		Large abscess may require
		  intubation while awake
		  (can lead to
		  parapharyngeal space)

*Infection in these areas can lead to Ludwig's angina (sensation of choking and suffocation). The majority of cases originate from tooth infection with approximately 75% originating from second or third molar.

■ Mobile tooth/teeth
■ Severe infection—trismus, dysphagia, airway compromise, and necrotizing fasciitis

Treatment

The treatment of dentoalveolar abscesses is dependent on the extent of the infection as well as the involvement of deep spaces. If the infection is localized and easily accessible, then it can be treated with either needle aspiration or incision and drainage. If the infection is more complex and widespread, involving the deep spaces, or the patient has respiratory compromise, then rapid referral to an oral surgeon and anticipation of a surgical intervention in the operating room should be done.

Special Considerations

■ Pediatric patients
  ■ Conscious sedation may be necessary for deep-seated or difficult-to-manage areas because of movement or severity
  ■ Each case should be considered independently
■ Patients who are immunocompromised or have comorbidities such as organ transplant, HIV-AIDS, diabetes, and/or cancer should be treated more aggressively and with a lower index of suspicion for abscess and infection
■ Patients with artificial heart valves and prosthetic joints should be prophylaxed based on the current American Heart Association/American College of Cardiology guidelines

Procedure Preparation

■ Topical anesthesia and injectable anesthesia (see Chapter 31)
■ Gauze
■ Nonsterile gloves
■ Kidney basin for patient to spit into
■ Culture swab for culture and sensitivity

NEEDLE ASPIRATION
■ 3- or 5-mL syringe
■ 21-gauge needle
■ Hydrogen peroxide and water (50:50 solution)

INCISION AND DRAINAGE
■ Hemostat
■ Scalpel (No. 11 or No. 15 blade)
■ Normal saline for irrigation
■ Packing material (1/4 inch gauze)
■ Fenestrated Penrose drain

Procedure

■ Dry oral mucosa
■ Apply topical anesthesia (see Chapter 31)
■ Perform either a local or nerve block (see Chapter 31)

NEEDLE ASPIRATION
- Insert needle into fluctuant area
- Aspirate
- Withdraw contents
- Obtain culture
- Have patient rinse the mouth with hydrogen peroxide and water

INCISION AND DRAINAGE (SEE CHAPTER 21 FOR ILLUSTRATIONS OF THE PROCEDURE)
- Make a small incision over the fluctuant area
  - Direct the point of the scalpel blade toward the alveolar surface
- Insert the tip of the hemostat into the incision
- Gently perform blunt dissection of the area to break up loculations
- Place the culture swab into the incision
- Irrigate with normal saline
  - Have the patient lean forward or to the side to prevent aspiration and choking
- Insert packing if the wound is large enough
  - You can suture the end of the packing to the mucosa with an absorbable suture to prevent aspiration

Some abscesses can extend from intraoral to extraoral and may need to be incised through the facial skin. Incision and drainage should be performed intraorally when at all possible to minimize scarring. If the abscess needs an extraoral approach, please follow the procedure for subcutaneous abscesses in Chapter 21.

Postprocedure Considerations

PAIN
- Pain medication should be prescribed based on the patient's pain level and tolerance
- Relieving the abscess can significantly reduce the pain

INFECTION
- Oral antibiotics should be prescribed (amoxicillin-clavulonate, clindamycin)

Educational Points

- Frequent warm salt water rinses for wounds without packing
- Proper intraoral hygiene and regular visits to the dentist are important for the prevention of further caries and infection
- Follow-up 1 to 2 days with either a dentist or oral surgeon

Complications

- Cavernous sinus thrombosis
- Fistula formation—chronic infection
- Ludwig's angina
- Maxillary sinusitis
- Osteomyelitis

DENTAL FRACTURE

Background

Dental trauma is commonly seen in office, urgent, and emergency care settings. The majority of injuries occur from contact sports but many occur from altercations, falls, or motor vehicle or motorcycle crashes. Fractures of the posterior teeth can occur from whiplash-type injury or striking of the chin closing jaw forcibly.

Many dental injuries can be accompanied by intraoral lacerations. Careful probing of the laceration is required to make sure chips and fragments are not in the laceration(s). If a tooth fragment cannot be located, radiographs need to be performed to rule out aspiration or ingestion of the tooth or large fragment.

Crown fractures can be classified as uncomplicated or complicated. The root fractures are difficult to diagnose and often require radiographs for definitive diagnosis and should always be referred to a dentist, orthodontist, or oral surgeon for prompt treatment and follow-up. Crown fractures can be placed in a three-category classification system known as the Ellis classification (Figure 32.1). Please see Table 32.2 for classification, presentation, and treatment of fractures.

Special Considerations

■ Children are at increased risk of infection with Ellis II and III fractures because of the increased pulp-to-dentin ratio. Dental referral should be within 24 hours of the injury
■ Patients who are immunocompromised are at increased risk for infection because of the decreased immune response. Antibiotic therapy and close follow-up is required with these patients

Procedure Preparation

■ Topical anesthesia and injectable anesthesia (see Chapter 31)
■ Gauze
■ Nonsterile gloves
■ Kidney basin for patient to spit
■ Calcium hydroxide, zinc oxide, or glass ionomer composites
■ Dental spatula
■ Tongue depressor (if dental spatula is not available for mixing the composite)
■ Cotton-tipped applicators (if dental spatula is not available for application onto tooth)

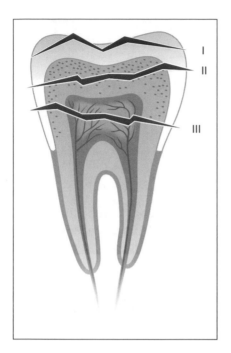

FIGURE 32.1 Ellis classification of tooth fracture.

TABLE 32.2 Ellis Classification of Crown Fractures

Ellis Class	Complicated or Uncomplicated	Fracture Location	Presentation	Treatment
Ellis I	Uncomplicated	Enamel	Sharp edges of tooth Little to no sensitivity	Smooth rough edges with emery board
Ellis II	Uncomplicated	Enamel Dentin	Sensitivity to temperature and air Yellow or pink tint to dentin	Supraperiosteal block Cap tooth with composite
Ellis III	Complicated	Enamel Dentin Pulp	Pain Dentin pink Frank bleeding	Supraperiosteal block Cap tooth with composite Immediate referral to dental specialist

- Aluminum foil*
- Emery board

Procedure

ELLIS I
- Smooth rough surface with emery board

ELLIS II AND ELLIS III
- Dry oral mucosa
- Apply topical anesthesia
- Perform either a local or nerve block
- Mix the catalyst and base of the composite material as directed on the label with the dental spatula (1:1 ratio)
  - A tongue depressor can be used in place of a spatula
- Dry the tooth using gauze (have the patient bite down on the gauze)
- Apply the mixture to the tooth with the dental spatula
- Allow the mixture to dry per the composite material instructions (usually a few minutes)

Postprocedure Considerations

ASPIRATION/INGESTION
- Tooth and tooth fragments have the potential to be swallowed or aspirated. Care should be given to avoid this

Educational Points

- Soft foods
- Avoid chewing on affected side/tooth
- Risk of pulp necrosis, color change, and/or root reabsorption with any fracture is a possibility

Complications

- Pulp death
- Decreased dental arch
- Ankylosis
- Color change
- Abscess
- Disruption of permanent tooth with fracture to primary tooth

---

AUTHOR'S PEARL

- *Reassure the patient to alleviate anxiety*

---

*Aluminum foil can be placed on top of a cap but is not necessary if referral to the dental specialist is within 24 hours.

SUBLUXATION AND LUXATION

Background

Dental trauma can result in a subluxation (i.e., mobile tooth or teeth), or luxation (i.e., partial or complete displacement of the tooth or teeth). Mobile or displaced teeth can be divided into four categories or types (Table 32.3).

Patient Presentation

■ Pain
■ Mobile tooth/teeth
■ Missing tooth/teeth
■ Bleeding

Treatment

The treatment of subluxation and luxation depends on the degree of mobility and extent of the injury. The goal of treatment is to secure the tooth in place as soon as possible and refer to the dentist within 24 hours of the injury. Pulp necrosis, color change, and necrosis of the alveolar ligaments can result from the trauma.

Subluxation of a primary tooth should not require any intervention unless the tooth is interfering with occlusion. The periodontal paste (Coe-Pak) can be used to secure a grossly mobile tooth/teeth until seen by a dental specialist within 24 hours. However, primary teeth that are a complete luxation (avulsion) should not be replaced in the socket.

A complete luxation of permanent tooth/teeth requires prompt attention and replacement of the tooth/teeth into the respective socket. The alveolar ligament cells

TABLE 32.3 Luxation Categories: Type, Mechanism, and Treatment

Type	Mechanism	Treatment
Extrusive	Tooth lifted up partially out of socket	Splint Dental referral
Intrusive	Tooth pushed down into the socket The apex of the tooth may be crushed or fractured	Radiographs Dental referral within 24 hours
Lateral	Tooth displaced laterally may be facial, lingual, or medial May be associated with alveolar wall injury	Splint Dental referral within 24 hours
Complete	Tooth forced completely out of socket Also known as avulsion	Supraperiosteal block Replace tooth in socket Splint or temporary suture Immediate dental referral Soft or liquid diet depending on severity and treatment Antibiotic prophylaxis

can begin to die as early as 60 minutes. The use of milk or commercial "save a tooth" preparations can increase this time significantly. If the preparations are not available to the patient, then the patient should be encouraged to place the tooth in mouth with his or her saliva.

The use of periodontal paste to splint the tooth/teeth into place as well as a temporary suture technique will be discussed in this section.

Contraindications and Relative Contraindications

- Fractured tooth
- Severe maxillofacial trauma/injury
- Extended period of time after complete luxation
- Contamination
- Special considerations
- Immunocompromised, diabetics

Procedure Preparation

REPLACING THE TOOTH/TEETH INTO THE SOCKET
- Gauze
- Absorbent pads
- Topical and supraperiosteal block materials (see Chapter 31)
- Frazier suction tip
- Suction apparatus
- Normal saline

SPLINTING
- Nonsterile gloves
- Gauze
- Lubricant
- Periodontal paste (Coe-Pak)

TEMPORARY SUTURE
- Suture kit
- Gauze
- Sterile gloves
- Absorbable suture material

Procedure

REPLACING THE TOOTH/TEETH INTO THE SOCKET
- Topical and supraperiosteal block (Chapter 31)
- Check the oral cavity for trauma (i.e., fracture)
- Gently suction the socket for blood clots, being careful not to suction the wall of the socket
- Irrigate the area with normal saline
- Gently rinse off the tooth holding it by the crown only
  - Never scrub or rub the tooth, especially the root
- Gently, but firmly, replace the tooth in the socket

■ The position does not have to be perfect but should be anatomically correct
■ Splint or suture if the tooth is too mobile after insertion

SPLINTING (FIGURE 32.2)

Grossly mobile or replaced tooth/teeth
■ Replace the tooth/teeth into the socket as described previously
■ Mix the periodontal paste per the instructions
  ■ Mix base with catalyst to make a moderately sticky paste
■ Completely dry the enamel and gingival with gauze
■ Place lubricant on gloved fingers
■ Place the paste over the affected tooth/teeth and the adjacent teeth
  ■ Be sure you apply the paste to the grooves between the teeth

TEMPORARY SUTURE (FIGURE 32.3)
■ Replace tooth/teeth into the socket as described previously
■ Insert the suture needle into the gingival at the border of the replaced tooth
■ Bring the suture straight down behind the tooth, coming out in front of the tooth

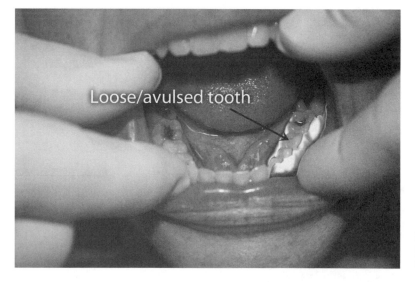

FIGURE 32.2 Securing loose-avulsed tooth with compound.

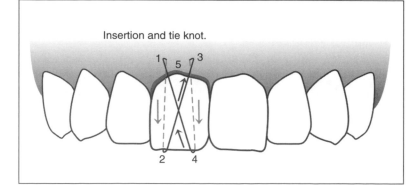

FIGURE 32.3 Temporary suture.

- Cross the tooth with the suture
- Insert the suture needle into the gingival on the opposite tooth border
- Bring the suture straight down behind the tooth, coming out in front of the tooth
- Cross the tooth with the suture
- Tie a square knot

Postprocedure Considerations

If the tooth/teeth do not remain in place or are too mobile with splinting, then the temporary suture technique should be used. The patient should be medicated for pain and prophylaxed with antibiotics (penicillin or clindamycin)

Educational Points

- Minimally mobile tooth/teeth
  - Soft diet
  - Dental specialist follow-up
- Grossly mobile or complete luxations
  - Liquid to soft diet
  - Dental specialist follow-up within 24 hours

Complications

- Loss of tooth/teeth
- Decreased dental arch
- Ankylosis
- Color change
- Abscess
- Disruption of permanent tooth with fracture to primary tooth

---

AUTHOR'S PEARL

- *Always be honest with the patient and/or parent about the potential outcome*

RESOURCES

Benko, R. (2010). Regional anesthesia of the head and neck. In J. R. Roberts & J. R. Hedges (Eds.), *Clinical procedures in emergency medicine*, (5th ed., pp. 1220–1225 & 1229–1233). Philadelphia: Saunders Elsevier.

Chow, A. W. (2010). Orofacial odontogenic infections. In G. L. Mandell, J. E. Bennett, & R. Dolin (Eds.), *Principles and practice of infectious diseases*. New York: Churchill and Livingstone. Retrieved from http://www.mdconsult.com/book/player/book.do?method= display&type=bookPage&decorator=header&eid=4-u1.0-B978-0-443-06839-3..00060-6–

s0040&displayedEid=4-u1.0-B978-0-443-06839-3..00060-6–s0045&uniq=188210824&
isbn=978-0-443-06839-3&sid=965655401#lpState=open&lpTab=contentsTab&content=
4-u1.0-B978-0-443-06839-3..00060-6%3Bfrom%3Dtoc%3Btype%3DbookPage%3Bisbn%
3D978-0-443-06839-3

Douglass, A. B., & Douglass, J. M. (2003). Common dental emergencies. *American Family Physician, 67*(3), 511–516.

Drezner, J. A., Harmon, K. G., & O'Kane, J. W. (2007). Sports trauma to the teeth, face and eye. In R. E. Rakel (Ed.), *Textbook of family medicine*, (7th ed.). Philadelphia: Saunders Elsevier. Retrieved from http://www.mdconsult.com/das/book/body/188210824-5/0/1481/482.html?tocnode=53394272&fromURL=482.html#4-u1.0-B978-1-4160-2467-5..50043-9–cesec26_2486

Hermann, H. J., & Laskin, D. M. (2007). In P. S. Auerbach (Ed.), *Wilderness medicine*, (5th ed.). Philadelphia: Mosby Elsevier. Retrieved from http://www.mdconsult.com/das/book/body/188210824-3/0/1483/238.html?tocnode=54235634&fromURL=238.html#4-u1.0-B978-0-323-03228-5..50031-8_1433

Kliegman, R. M., Behrman, R. E., Jenson, H. B., & Stanton, B. F. (Eds.) (2007). Dental trauma. In *Nelson textbook of pediatrics*, (18th ed.). Philadelphia: Saunders. Retrieved from http://www.mdconsult.com/das/book/body/188210824-8/965665260/1608/772.html#4-u1.0-B978-4160-2450-7..50313-3_6366

Matijevic, S., Lazic, Z., Kuljic-Kapulica, N., & Nonkovic, Z. (2009). Empirical antimicrobial therapy of acute dentoalveolar abscess. *Vojnosanitetski Pregled: Military medical & Pharmaceutical Journal of Serbia, 66*(7), 544–550.

Nguyen, D. H., & Martin, J. T. (2008). Common dental infections in the primary care setting. *American Family Physician, 77*(6), 797–802, 806.

Peng, L. F., Kazzi, A. A., Peng, W., & Cheng, C. (2009). Dental, fractured tooth. Retrieved from http://emedicine.medscape.com/article/763458-overview and http://emedicine.medscape.com/article/763458-treatment

Peng, L. F., Kazzi, A. A., Peng, W., & Cheng, C. (2009). Dental, avulsed tooth. Retrieved from http://emedicine.medscape.com/article/763291-overview&and http://emedicine.medscape.com/article/763291-treatment

Peng, L. F., Kazzi, A. A., Peng, W., & Cheng, C. (2008). Dental, displaced tooth. Retrieved from http://emedicine.medscape.com/article/763378-overview and http://emedicine.medscape.com/article/763378-treatment

Procedure for Arthrocentesis

KEITH A. LAFFERTY

BACKGROUND

Joints allow free movement between two bone surfaces, which causes friction and generates heat. The cartilaginous articular surfaces (composed of collagen and proteoglycan substances) at the end of bones are highly compressible and well lubricated by synovial fluid, which is secreted by cells of the synovial membrane lining the joint space which helps dissipate heat and allow smooth motion of the joint. These cells also participate in the inflammatory cascade and contain lysosomes in their cytoplasm. The high concentration of hyaluronic acid in the synovium gives it its high viscosity. Finally, a capsule encircles the entire joint, which is further supported by its surrounding ligaments, tendons, and muscle. The synovial membrane, periosteum, and joint capsule are rich in sensory nerve fibers. Of note, polymorphonuclear cells release hyaluronidase from their lysosomes, which enzymatically destroy hyaluronic acid, thereby decreasing the synovial fluid viscosity in inflammatory joint conditions. This thinning of the synovial fluid can be tested grossly by placing the drawn synovial fluid between the gloved thumb and index finger and, upon separating the fingers, measuring the fluid length, otherwise known as the string sign (Figure 33.1).

The inflamed joint can be a diagnostic challenge to even the most experienced provider. Furthermore, the clinical signs and symptoms that distinguish septic arthritis from other arthritides can have much overlap. Besides diagnostic reasons, arthrocentesis can be a therapeutic benefit providing relief from traumatic hemarthrosis and chronic arthritides.

DIFFERENTIAL DIAGNOSIS

- Cellulitis
- Bursitis
- Tendonitis
- Baker's cyst
- Deep vein thrombosis

PATIENT PRESENTATION

- Pain
- Swelling
- Possible erythema

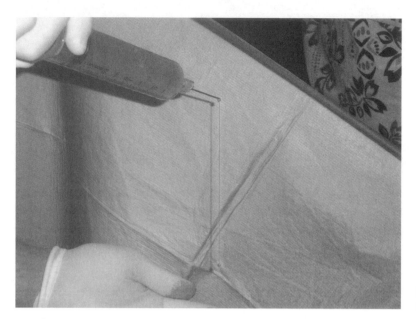

FIGURE 33.1 String sign.

TREATMENT

Clothing should be removed and the affected joint exposed. Aspirate as much fluid as possible for diagnostic and therapeutic reasons. It is paramount to rule out septic arthritis. The approach for arthrocentesis usually is the extensor surfaces which are secondary to most neurovascular structures that reside on the flexor surfaces, as well as larger joint exposure, being more superficial.

Fluid analysis should consist of a Gram stain and culture, cell count, and crystals. Note that a negative Gram stain does not rule out septic arthritis. In general, cell counts more than 50,000 WBCs/mm³ warrant treatment for septic arthritis. Gout and pseudogout have crystal formation and usually induce less than 50,000 WBCs/mm³. However, up to 20% of these arthrotides can induce a WBC count >50,000 WBCs/mm³. Rheumatoid arthritis and the seronegative arthritides also have usually induce less than 50,000/WBCs/mm³. Osteoarthritis has less than 4,000 WBCs/mm³.

CONTRAINDICATIONS

- Overlying cellulitis

RELATIVE CONTRAINDICATIONS

- Bleeding
- Diatheses
- Bacteremia
- Prosthetic joint

PROCEDURE PREPARATION

- Protective gown and sterile gloves
- Sterile drapes

- Skin cleanser with chlorhexidine or providone iodine
- Local anesthetic agent
- 10- to 60-mL syringe depending on joint size
- 18- to 22-gauge needle depending on joint size
- Red, purple, and green test tubes for lab analysis
- Sterile technique is mandatory and aseptic technique is paramount

PROCEDURE

Knee

- Position towels under the knee to give 15° of slight flexion
- For the medial approach, identify the medial midpatellar area; the site of entry should be just below this
- Direct a 18-gauge needle slightly cephalic toward the intercondylar femoral notch (Figure 33.2)
- Keep it just under the posterior surface of the patella
- Make sure that needle stays parallel to the floor
- A lateral approach may be done as well

Radiohumeral Joint (Elbow)

- Patient should be sitting upright in bed
- Elbow flexed at 90° on the table with the forearm in pronation
- Identify the lateral epicondyle and the head of the radius
- Using a 22-gauge needle, enter the joint in a medial matter, perpendicular to the joint (Figure 33.3)

Radiocarpal Joint (Wrist)

- Patient should be sitting upright in bed
- Forearm/wrist prone on the table with the wrist flexed at 30° with slight traction

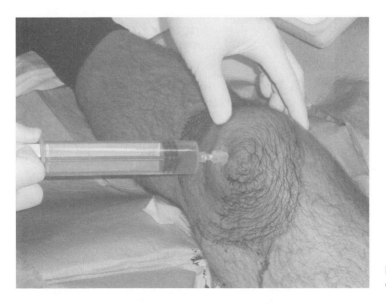

FIGURE 33.2 Knee arthrocentesis.

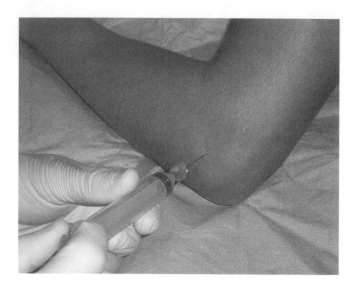

FIGURE 33.3 Radiohumeral arthrocentesis.

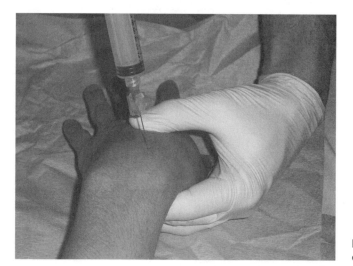

FIGURE 33.4 Radiocarpal arthrocentesis.

- Identify the dorsal radial tubercle (it is a prominence of the distal dorsal radius)
- The extensor pollicis longus tendon runs radial to this tubercle and also makes the dorsal tendon border the snuff box
- Enter the joint space with a 22-gauge needle distal to the radial tubercle and on the ulna side of the extensor pollicis longus tendon, where a sulcus can be palpated perpendicular to the skin (Figure 33.4)

Tibiatalar Joint (Ankle)

- Patient should be supine on the bed
- Foot in plantar flexion
- Identify the medial malleolar sulcus (lateral to the medial malleolus)

- The lateral margin of the sulcus is bordered by the anterior tibial tendon (best seen by active dorsiflexion)
- Insert a 20- or 22-gauge needle dorsally (perpendicular to the fibular shaft) into the medial malleolar sulcus (Figure 33.5)

Glenohumeral Joint (Shoulder)

- Patient should be sitting on stretcher with hands on their lap
- Identify the coracoid process medially and the humeral head laterally
- Insert a 20- or 22-gauge needle in the sulcus bordered by the coracoid and the humeral head
- Needle is inserted inferiorly and laterally to the coracoid and directed posteriorly (Figure 33.6)

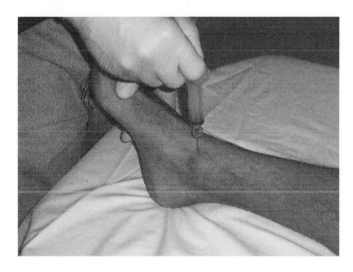

FIGURE 33.5 Tibiatalar arthrocentesis.

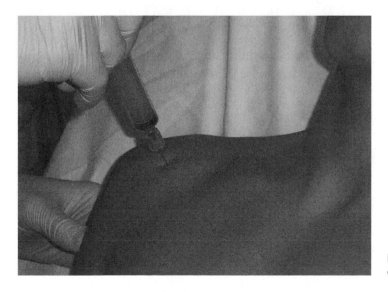

FIGURE 33.6 Glenohumeral arthrocentesis.

COMPLICATIONS

- Infection
- Hemarthrosis
- Corticosteroid related complications

AUTHOR'S PEARLS

- *Active and passive range of motion will always elicit pain in articular disease while rarely being elicited in periarticular disease*
- *Relaxation of muscles is of paramount importance because their contraction narrows the joint surface*
- *Fat globules in the synovial fluid are diagnostic of a fracture*
- *Arthrocentesis of the acute traumatic hemarthrosis not only provides symptomatic relief of pain, but also allows proper assessment of ligamentous stability*
- *A dry tap is rare and one should question the proper position of the needle*
- *If minimal fluid returns, synovial culture trumps other lab tests*
- *Ultrasound guidance may be of benefit in localizing difficult joint spaces*
- *Because of the action of hyaluronidase on hyaluronic acid, viscosity can be tested by dripping a small amount of fluid from the syringe needle and measuring the length of the string created. In inflammatory conditions, especially in infectious etiologies, the "string sign" will be much less than 10 cm*
- *Note that extracapsular disease can mimic articular diseases such as bursitis, tendonitis, and cellulitis*

RESOURCES

Lowery, D. W. (2006). Arthritis. In J. Marx, R. Hockberger, & R. Walls (Eds.), *Rosen's emergency medicine concepts and clinical practice* (pp. 1780–1781). Philadelphia: Mosby, Elsevier.

Ma, L., Cranney, A., & Holroyd-Leduc, J. M. (2009). Acute monoarthritis: What is the cause of my patient's painful swollen joint? *Canadian Medical Association Journal, 180*(1), 59–65.

Parrillo, S. J., & Fisher, J. (2004). Arthrocentesis. In J. Roberts & J. Hedges (Eds.), *Clinical procedures in emergency medicine* (pp. 1042–1056). Philadelphia: Saunders Elsevier.

Siva, C. (2003). Diagnosing acute monoarthritis in adults: A practical approach for the family physician. *American Family Physician, 68*(1), 83–90.

Wise, C. (2008). Arthrocentesis and injection of joints and soft tissue. In G. S. Firestein, E. D. Harris, R. C. Budd, I. B. McInnes, & S. Buddy (Eds.), *Firestein: Kelley's textbook of rheumatology.* Philadelphia: W. B. Saunders Company.

34

Procedure for Therapeutic Joint Injection

Keith A. Lafferty

BACKGROUND

This modality has been used since the 1950s and its use has been increasing in recent years. Injured joint tissue leads to a proliferation of the inflammatory cascade, in part from the synovial cells themselves and also from circulating polymorphonuclear leukocytes. This proliferation of cytokines increases blood flow, induces pain and swelling, and decreases range of motion. Corticosteroids suppress this inflammatory cascade by decreasing capillary permeability and by attenuating many of the cytokine effects.

The ideal steroid for injection should have a long duration of activity, have little or no postinjection pain, and should possess minimal side effects. Different agents have not been studied in a comparable manner. The duration of the effect is related to the solubility of the agent, with lower solubility corticosteroids having an increased joint duration. Because long-acting agents are in a crystalline solution, they can cause a postinjection flare that does not occur when using a short-acting solution. Combining two such agents together offsets each other's shortcomings. Also, mixing the solution with a long-acting anesthetic agent provides even earlier relief of symptoms and dilutes the solution. Also, in general, larger joints require more corticosteroids than smaller joints (up to 10 mL should be instilled into the knee joint) (Figure 34.1).

PATIENT PRESENTATION

- Pain
- Tenderness
- Swelling
- Erythema
- Decreased range of motion

TREATMENT (Table 34.1)

Only after aspiration of synovial fluid and positively ruling out septic arthritis, therapeutic joint injection may be implemented. Basically any arthritic condition, except septic arthritis, is a candidate for this treatment modality such as, but not limited to, osteo, rheumatoid, gout, pseudogout, and autoimmune arthrotides.

TABLE 34.1 Summary of Treatment for Therapeutic Joint Infection

	Large Joint (mg)	Small Joint (mg)	Potency	Solubility	Duration
Hydrocortosone acetate (Hydrocortone)	NA	NA	1	High	Low
Triamcinolone acetonide (Kenalog)	20	2–6	5	Intermediate	Intermediate
Triamcinolone hexacetonide (Aristospan)	20	2–6	5	Intermediate	Intermediate
Methylprednisolone acetate (Depo-Medrol)	40	3.5–10.5	5	Intermediate	Intermediate
Betamethasone acetate/sodium phosphate (Celestone Soluspan)	6	1.5–3	25	Low	High
Dexamethasone acetate (Decadron-La)	5	0.5–1.5	25	Low	High

CONTRAINDICATIONS

- An infection of either articular or overlying periarticular tissue
- Acute fractures
- Prosthetic joints

RELATIVE CONTRAINDICATIONS

- Bleeding diathesis
- Bacteremia
- Chronic debilitating diseases such as tuberculosis
- Achilles/patella tendonopathies
- Two previous injections with failure

PROCEDURE PREPARATION

- See arthrocentesis on particular joints in Chapter 33
- Sterile gloves
- Sterile drapes
- Skin cleanser with chlorhexidine or providone iodine
- Local anesthetic agent
- 5- to 10-cc syringe depending on joint size

■ 18- to 22-gauge needle depending on joint size

■ Sterile technique is mandatory and aseptic technique is paramount

PROCEDURE

Occasionally, a therapeutic joint injection immediately follows an arthrocentesis. In this situation, an angiocath may be used with the catheter left in place after the arthrocentesis. The corticosteroid-filled syringe can now be attached to the catheter and injection procedures may be followed (Figure 34.1). To view figures corresponding with anatomical landmarks, see Chapter 33.

Knee

■ Position towels under the knee to give 15° of slight flexion

■ For the medial approach, identify the medial midpatellar area; the site of entry should be just below this

■ Direct a 20-gauge needle slightly cephalic toward the intercondylar femoral notch

■ Keep the needle just under the posterior surface of the patella

■ Make sure the needle stays parallel to the floor

■ A lateral approach may be done as well

Radiohumeral Joint (Elbow)

■ Patient should be sitting upright in bed

■ Elbow flexed at 90° on the table with the forearm in pronation

■ Identify the lateral epicondyle and the head of the radius

■ Using a 22-gauge needle, enter the joint in a medial manner, perpendicular to the joint

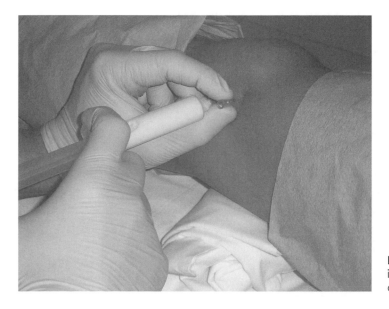

FIGURE 34.1 Steroid joint injection using an angio-catheter.

Radiocarpal Joint (Wrist)

- Patient should be sitting upright in bed
- Forearm/wrist prone on the table with the wrist flexed at 30° with slight traction
- Identify the dorsal radial tubercle (it is a prominence of the distal dorsal radius)
- The extensor pollicis longus tendon runs radial to this tubercle and also makes the dorsal tendon border the snuff box
- Enter the joint space with a 22-gauge needle distal to the radial tubercle and on the ulna side of the extensor pollicis longus tendon where a sulcus can be palpated perpendicular to the skin

Tibiatalar Joint (Ankle)

- Patient should be supine on the bed
- Foot in plantar flexion
- Identify the medial malleolar sulcus (lateral to the medial malleolus)
- The lateral margin of the sulcus is bordered by the anterior tibial tendon (best seen by active dorsiflexion)
- Insert a 20- or 22-gauge needle dorsally (perpendicular to the fibular shaft) into the medial malleolar sulcus

Glenohumeral Joint (Shoulder)

- Patient should be sitting on a stretcher with hands on his or her lap
- Identify the coracoid process medially and the humeral head laterally
- Insert a 20- or 22-gauge needle in the sulcus bordered by the coracoid and the humeral head
- Insert the needle inferiorly and laterally to the coracoid and directed posteriorly

COMPLICATIONS

- Infection
- Subcutaneous atrophy and calcification
- Tendon rupture (repeated injections)
- Juxta-articular bone necrosis (repeated injections)
- Intra-articular bleeding
- Transient steroid flare

AUTHOR'S PEARLS

- *If there is any suspicion of septic arthritis, abandon this treatment*
- *Ultrasound guidance has been shown to improve intra-articular needle position, and hence improve the outcome*
- *Limit injections to a span of 3 months apart*

RESOURCES

Carek, P. J., & Hunter, M. H. (2005). Joint and soft tissue injections in primary care. *Clinics in Family Practice, 7*(2), 359–378.

Lavelle, W., Lavelle, E. D., & Lavelle, L. Intra-articular injections. *Medical Clinics of North America, 91*(2), 241–250.

Stephens, M., & Beutler, A. (2008). Musculoskeletal injections: A review of the evidence. *American Family Physician, 78*(8), 971–976.

Wise, C. (2008). Arthrocentesis and injection of joints and soft tissue. In G. Firestein (Ed.), *Firestein: Kelley's textbook of rheumatology.* Philadelphia: W. B. Saunders Company; accessed from http://www.mdconsult.com/das/book/body/217633773-3/1049214966/1807/344.html #4-u1.0-B978-1-4160-3285-4..10049-X_1409

35

Procedure for Shoulder Dislocation

KEITH A. LAFFERTY

BACKGROUND

Because the glenohumeral joint has the greatest range of motion of any joint in the body, it also is the most commonly dislocated joint. Contributing to this is an inately loose capsule, shallow glenoid fossa, lack of anterior muscular support, and a relatively thin anterior inferior glenohumeral ligament, which is prone to tears. Shoulder dislocations are divided into anterior and posterior based on the position of the humeral head in relation to the glenoid fossa. Note that posterior dislocations occur 2% of the time and will only be briefly discussed. Anterior subluxations are subdivided into subcoracoid (most common), subglenoid (together these two represent 99% of all anterior dislocations), subclavicular, and intrathoracic (Figures 35.1 and 35.2).

The mechanism of injury is usually an indirect force of abduction, extension, and external rotation. Rarely it is the result of a direct blow to the shoulder. In general, sporting activity in the young and falling in the elderly are the culprits. Patients less than 30 years of age have more than 80% recurrence rate, whereas those more than 40 years of age have a much lower recurrence rate (10%). Studies have shown an increase in the incidence of anterior inferior glenohumeral ligament avulsions from the glenoid rim, now thought to be the primary factor for recurrent dislocations; it is amenable to arthroscopic surgical repair. In fact, the current evidence suggests that younger athletic patients who are unwilling to modify their activities may benefit from stabilization after their initial dislocation to avoid recurrent instability. Also, rotator cuff injuries are much more common and are reported in up to 15% in those who are more than 40 years of age as these tendons weaken as one ages. Axillary nerve injury in the form of neuropraxia from nerve traction is the most common neuronal injury and the patient almost always returns to full function.

Associated fractures are common and are reported in up to 50% of cases, giving importance to preprocedural x-rays. Compression fracture of the humeral head caused by its impingement on the inferior glenoid rim causes the most common fracture, known as the Hill-Sachs deformity. A corresponding fracture of this deformity of the inferior glenoid rim, known as the Bankart lesion, also occurs via the same mechanism. The greater tuberosity is also susceptible to an avulsion type fracture. None of these fractures change treatment.

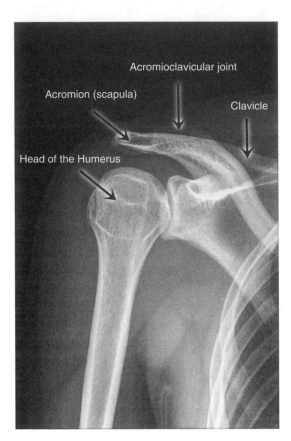

Acromioclavicular joint

Acromion (scapula)

Clavicle

Head of the Humerus

FIGURE 35.1 Normal shoulder joint.

PATIENT PRESENTATION

- Severe pain
- Injured extremity held by the contralateral arm with slight external rotation and abduction
- The normal rounded contour of the shoulder is flattened with a shelflike appearance, secondary to a now-prominent acromian process (Figure 35.3)
- Anterior shoulder appears full
- Patient is unable to use the ipsilateral hand to palpate the contralateral shoulder, otherwise known as the scarf sign

Reduction Techniques

Regardless of the technique used, the astute clinician should be familiar with multiple techniques as no technique carries a 100% success rate. Also, the literature is lacking in comparative studies in comparison techniques. In general, conscious sedation is recommended with the exception of the recurrent dislocation presenting immediately. Basically all techniques involve a form of traction, leverage, or scapular manipulation. Essentially one is either moving the humeral head with the glenoid fossa remaining fixed or vice versa.

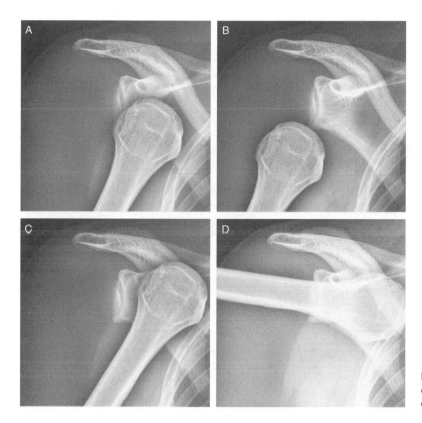

FIGURE 35.2 Types of anterior shoulder dislocations.

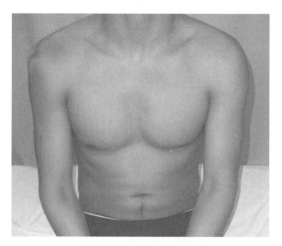

FIGURE 35.3 Anterior shoulder dislocation.

CONTRAINDICATIONS

■ In patients with a contraindication to sedation, such as intoxicated patients, intra-articular anesthetic injection may be beneficial (see Chapter 34)
■ Open dislocations

PROCEDURE PREPARATION/REDUCTION TECHNIQUE

- Prepare for conscious sedation (cardiac monitor, pulse oximeter, etc.)
- Assistant
- Two sheets

PROCEDURE

Modified Traction-Countertraction

- Patient is supine with the arm abducted and elbow flexed at 90°
- Tie and wrap a sheet around the waist of the provider with the other end placed in the anticub fossa of the patient at the flexed elbow
- An assistant has another sheet wrapped across the chest of the patient at the level of the axillae, applying countertraction (Figure 35.4)
- The provider leans back (traction) and rotates the arm externally and possibly internally at the same time
- Pressure applied to the head of the humerus may facilitate this technique

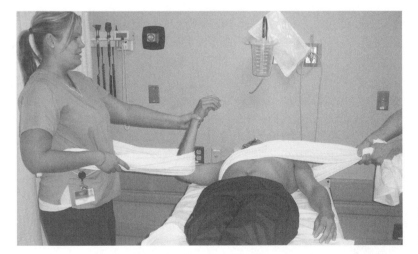

FIGURE 35.4 Modified traction-counter-traction method.

External Rotation

- Patient is supine with the arm adducted to the side
- Gradually the elbow is flexed to 90° while slow forearm external rotation is applied until the arm lies in the coronal plane (Figure 35.5)
- This should take place slowly, usually more than 10 minutes
- A clunk sound may not be appreciated by the provider or the patient
- This technique may be attempted without sedation in the appropriate patient
- Also of benefit, this technique requires only one provider

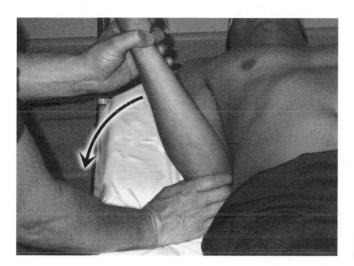

FIGURE 35.5 External rotation method.

Scapula Manipulation

Reduction is accomplished by repositioning the glenoid fossa rather than the humeral head.

■ The patient is placed in the prone position
■ Traction is applied on the ipsilateral arm, which is hanging off the bed, with the help of weights or an assistant
■ The provider pushes the inferior tip of the scapula with two thumbs medially and superiorly while stabilizing the superior scapula with the top hand, which causes the glenoid to move anteriorly and caudal to meet the humeral head
■ This technique may be attempted without sedation in the appropriate patient
■ This can be difficult in heavier patients as landmarks are diminished

POSTPROCEDURE CONSIDERATIONS

■ Typically, after reduction, all patients should be placed in a sling and swathe and should follow-up with orthopedics
■ Note that current evidence suggests that the immobilization of a first-time traumatic shoulder dislocation in external rotation for 3 weeks reduces the risk of recurrent dislocation as compared to standard internal rotation immobilization
■ Proper analgesics should be given
■ Although most provider perform x-rays after reduction, if the patient displays stability of the joint with a normal neurological exam, and is able to take the ipsilateral hand and touch the contralateral shoulder, x-rays may be forgone

AUTHOR'S PEARLS

- *Younger patients usually redislocate, older patients usually do not*
- *Older patients may injure their rotator cuff tendons, younger patients usually do not*
- *Posterior dislocations are often missed radiographically. A "Y" view will show the humeral head posterior to the glenoid fossa*
- *Gradual, gentle traction and rotation, along with maximal muscular rotation, are the cornerstones to successful reduction techniques*
- *Avoid jerking forces because this increases complications and decreases success rates*
- *If a patient can take the ipsilateral hand and touch the contralateral shoulder (scarf sign), there is no dislocation (Figure 35.6)*
- *Ultrasound is being used more often to complement clinical confirmation of dislocation and adequate reduction*

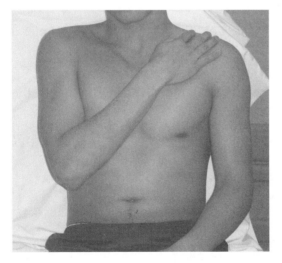

FIGURE 35.6 Scarf sign.

RESOURCES

Dodson, C. C., & Cordasco, F. A. (2008). Anterior glenohumeral joint dislocations. *Orthopedic Clinics of North America, 39*(4), 507–518.

Halberg, M. J. (2009). Bedside ultrasound for verification of shoulder reduction. *American Journal of Emergency Medicine, 27*(1), 503–504.

Hendey, G. W. (2000). Necessity of radiographs in the emergency department management of shoulder dislocations. *Annals of Emergency Medicine, 36*(2), 108–113.

McNeil, N. J. (2009). Postreduction management of first-time traumatic anterior shoulder dislocations. *Annals of Emergency Medicine, 53*(6), 811–813.

Newton, E. J. (2007). Emergency department management of selected orthopedic injuries. *Emergency Medicine Clinics of North America, 25*(3), 763–793.

Ufberg, J., & McNamara, R. (2004). Management of common dislocations. In J. Roberts & J. Hedges (Eds.), *Clinical procedures in emergency medicine* (pp. 948–960). Philadelphia: Saunders Elsevier.

Procedure for Patella Dislocation

KEITH A. LAFFERTY

BACKGROUND

Mechanism of injury usually involves twisting with an externally rotated knee. Most often the patella is displaced laterally over the lateral condyle of the femur. Medial and superior dislocations are rare and may require surgical repair. In order for the patella to be displaced laterally, there must be a tear of the medial patella retinaculum. The typical case involves an adolescent in a sport that requires a sudden knee extension, external rotation, and valgus maneuver, which is essentially a cutting maneuver of the athlete such as in hockey and gymnastics. Although less common, dislocation can result via a direct blow to the anterior medial patella. Fifteen percent of patients have recurrent dislocations.

Do not confuse a patella dislocation with a femur-tibia (knee) dislocation. Interestingly enough, this is more common in females and up to 24% display a family history. A true knee dislocation is an absolute emergency and presents spontaneously reduced half of the time. There is a high morbidity, as up to 30% of cases have an associated popliteal arterial injury.

PATIENT PRESENTATION

- Obvious laterally displaced patella (Figure 36.1)
- Sometimes tenting of the skin with the knee in mild flexion
- Inability to ambulate

TREATMENT

Closed reduction can occur spontaneously. X-rays are not routinely required for prereduction but may be done at postreduction to detect osteochondral fractures, which are reported to be as high as 50%, although most are identified by arthroscopy. Sedation is rarely required.

PROCEDURE

- Patient should be lying in the supine position
- Apply active knee extension while applying anterior-medial pressure to the lateral edge of the patella (Figure 36.2)

POSTPROCEDURE CONSIDERATIONS

- A knee immobilizer should be used for 3 to 6 weeks in order for the medial patella retinaculum to heal
- Patients with recurrent dislocations may require an arthroscopic release of the lateral retinaculum to blunt its pulling force on the patella laterally

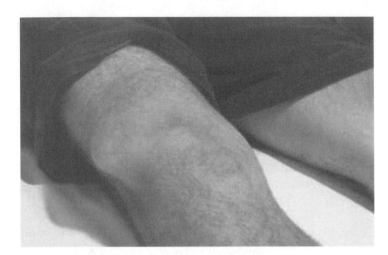

FIGURE 36.1 Patella dislocation.

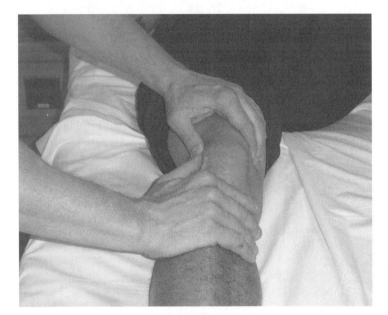

FIGURE 36.2 Patella dislocation—closed reduction.

AUTHOR'S PEARLS

- *Reduction can often be done while the patient is on the EMS stretcher*
- *If the reduction is unsuccessful, the medial facet of the patella may be locked on the lateral femoral condyle, which will require downward pressure on the lateral edge of the patella*
- *Patients presenting with complete ligamentous disruption of the knee without a deformity should be suspected of having a spontaneous knee dislocation and should be treated as such*

RESOURCES

Andrish, J. (2008). The management of recurrent patellar dislocation. *Orthopedic Clinics of North America, 39*(3), 313–327.

Arendt, E. A. (2002). Current concepts of lateral patella dislocation. *Clinics of Sports Medicine, 21*(3), 499–519.

Dlabach, J. A. (2007). Acute dislocations of the patella. In T. S. Canale (Ed.), *Campbell's operative orthopedics*. Retrieved from http://www.mdconsult.com/das/book/body/192201420-10/976162489/1584/422.html#4-u1.0-B978-0-323-03329-9..50060-X–cesec4_3265

Geiderman, J. M. (2006). General principles of orthopedic injuries. In J. Marx, R. Hockberger, & R. Walls (Eds.), *Rosen's emergency medicine concepts and clinical practice* (Vol. X; pp. 564–565, 784–786). Philadelphia: Mosby Elsevier.

Procedure for Digit Dislocation

Keith A. Lafferty

BACKGROUND

Because of the high exposure of the hand, injuries are common, especially among athletes. A basic review of the articular anatomy is key to understanding and treating these common injuries.

The anatomic structure of the proximal interphalangeal (PIP), distal interphalangeal (DIP), and metacarpophalangeal (MCP) joints are fundamentally the same. Note that, however, the MCP joint is condyloid in shape allowing some abduction and adduction, whereas the PIP/DIP joints are more of hinge or tongue and groove joints, which do not allow lateral movement. The ligamentous support of the MCP joints are thicker and are also reinforced by the deep transverse metacarpal ligament and hence are much less prone to injury.

The MCP/interphalangeal (IP) joints are stabilized laterally by the strong collateral ligaments and the flexor surface is supported by the vulnerable volar plate ligament (Figure 37.1). The extensor hood complex helps prevent volar dislocation. Because of this lateral-volar support, dorsal dislocations are more common and also, by definition, imply a disruption of the volar plate. Lateral dislocations have a disruption of one of the collateral ligaments and at least a partial tear of the volar plate. Dislocations are more common at the PIP joint than at the DIP joint secondary to the additional stability of the flexor and extensor tendon insertions at the distal phalanx.

Mechanistically, the usual forces are that of an axial load injury with hyperextension, with subsequent tearing of the volar plate and plus-or-minus collateral ligament injury. Interphalangeal dislocations occur in the toe with the same axial load and hyperextension mechanistic forces that apply to the fingers.

Classification of dislocated MCP/IP joints is either simple or complex. Simple implies that no soft tissue (volar plate, tendon) is interposed or entrapped in the joint, allowing an easy closed reduction. Complex implies there is soft tissue entrapment in the joint, making a closed reduction nearly impossible and the probable need for operative repair. Many MCP dislocations are of the complex variety.

The first MCP joint is much more susceptible than the other MCP joints for injury, most importantly involving the ulna collateral ligament. This is known as a "game keepers thumb." The integrity of this ligament is crucial for proper thumb opposition and normal grasping features of the hand. The patient may present with only localized tenderness along the ulna collateral ligament at the first MCP joint.

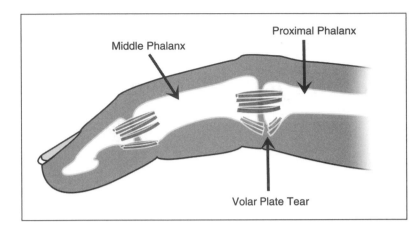

FIGURE 37.1 Volar and collateral ligament anatomy.

Associated volar plate injuries are common. Early recognition of this injury through ulna collateral stress testing is key in identifying such an injury. Proper immobilization and immediate orthopedic follow-up decreases morbidity. Skiers are susceptible to such injury, falling on an upright ski pole.

PATIENT PRESENTATION

Symptoms present as follows:

■ Acute pain
■ Swelling
■ Deformity (Figure 37.2)
■ Decreased range of motion

TREATMENT

Anesthesia can be performed using either a digital or metacarpal block for DIP/PIP dislocations or a wrist block (radial or ulna) for MCP dislocations. Closed reduction can be accomplished in most cases. Radiographs, before and after reduction, are used to identify fractures and confirm adequate reduction (Figure 37.3). The proper

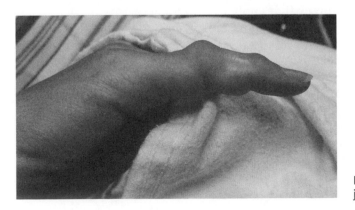

FIGURE 37.2 Digit dislocation—PIP joint.

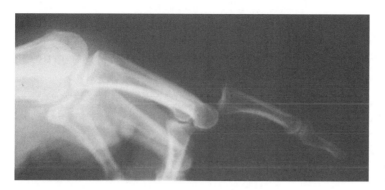

FIGURE 37.3 X-ray of dorsal PIP joint dislocation.

use of a methodical technique is paramount for successful reduction and, furthermore, to avoid causing a simple dislocation to become a complex one.

Open PIP/DIP dislocations should be reduced, copiously irrigated, sutured, and have immediate follow-up with orthopedics. Open MCP dislocations should be reduced, irrigated, and dressed, and then admitted for formal operative repair.

PROCEDURE PREPARATION

■ Patient should be comfortable with the dislocated joint well exposed
■ Local anesthetic agent
■ Rubber gloves
■ Finger splint, thumb spica, or buddy tape

PROCEDURE

PIP/DIP Closed Reduction

■ Exaggerate the deformity followed by hyperextension, longitudinal traction, and finally dorsal pressure (Figure 37.4)

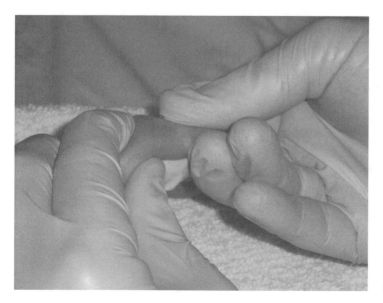

FIGURE 37.4 Closed reduction of PIP joint dislocation.

MCP Closed Reduction

This has an increased difficulty compared to IP reduction and a higher chance of complex dislocations. If an improper method is used, the chance of converting a simple dislocation to a complex dislocation is increased.

- Flex wrist in order to relax the stabilizing effects of the flexor tendons
- Extend and apply longitudinal traction
- Apply dorsal pressure
- Unlike IP reductions, excessive hyperextension and excessive longitudinal traction should be avoided

POSTPROCEDURE CONSIDERATIONS

- Postreduction radiographs are not necessary for uncomplicated reductions
- DIP splints are applied with the DIP and PIP joint in 20° of flexion
- PIP reductions should be splinted or buddy taped with treatment for 2 to 3 weeks
- Finger reductions should be splinted or buddy taped with treatment for 10 to 14 days
- First MCP dislocations are treated with a thumb spika and 20° of flexion for 4 weeks and immediate orthopedic follow-up
- Other MCP joint reductions are treated in flexion using a volar splint for 3 to 4 weeks
- Treatment of toe reductions is with buddy tape and a walking shoe for 2 to 3 weeks for the first toe and 10 to 14 days for the lesser toes

COMPLICATIONS

- Fractures
- Conversion of a simple dislocation into a complex one

AUTHOR'S PEARLS

- *Always remove rings from patients*
- *Volar dislocations are rare and often require operative repair*
- *Avoid long-term immobilization to eliminate the possible sequelae of joint stiffness and loss of flexion*
- *A firm grip can be ensured if the provider wears a tight rubber glove*
- *Upon reduction, always exaggerate the deformity first in order to lessen further injury and maximize successful reduction*
- *Because extrinsic flexors of both IP joints are four times stronger that their extensor counterparts, proper range of motion is mandatory in post-reduction care to prevent flexion contractures*

RESOURCES

Geiderman, J. M. (2006). General principles of orthopedic injuries. In J. Marx, R. Hockberger, & R. Walls (Eds.), *Rosen's emergency medicine concepts and clinical practice* (Vol. X; pp. 564–565, 784–786). Philadelphia: Mosby, Elsevier.

Leggit, J. C. (2006). Acute finger injuries: Part II. Fractures, dislocations, and thumb injuries. *American Family Physician, 73*(5), 827–834.

Polansky, R., & Kwon, N. S. (2009). Joint reduction, finger dislocation. Retrieved from http://emedicine.medscape.com/article/109206-overview

Ufberg, J., & McNamara, R. (2004). Management of common dislocations. In J. Roberts & J. Hedges (Eds.), *Clinical procedures in emergency medicine* (pp. 948–960). Philadelphia: Saunders Elsevier.

Young, G. M. (2008). Dislocation, interphalangeal: Differential diagnosis & workup. Retrieved from http://emedicine.medscape.com/article/823676-diagnosis

Procedure for Managing Nurse Maid's Elbow

Keith A. Lafferty

BACKGROUND

The typical presenting age of nurse maid's elbow is usually 1 to 3 years, with the most common being just over 2 years of age. There are cases in the literature of children from 6 months of age and up to 7 years of age with this condition, although this is rare. The typical mechanism is that of a sudden longitudinal traction of the arm with the elbow extended and slight pronation in the forearm. It is typically in the left arm as most care givers are right handed. Physiologically, the annular ligament stretches and tears at its attachment on the radial neck and slips between capetellum and the head of the radius. Note that 22% of patients report a fall and the recurrence rate is 20%.

PATIENT PRESENTATION

■ Patient cannot perform supination
■ Arm is noted to be in pronation of the wrist and slight flexion of the elbow (Figure 38.1)
■ The child is in no distress
■ Swelling, ecchymosis, and deformity are absent (unlike a fracture)
■ There may or may not be mild nonpoint tenderness
■ Resistance to supination

TREATMENT

For the most part, the treatment of nurse maid's elbow does not require a radiographic examination. Even when the history is vague, if the classic clinical presentation is confronted with an absence of point tenderness or swelling and a nondistressed child, a reduction may be done.

CONTRAINDICATIONS

■ Suspicion of a fracture, septic arthritis, tumor, or osteomyelitis

PROCEDURE PREPARATION

■ Have the child sit on the parent's lap
■ Parent holds the ipsilateral humerus in adduction

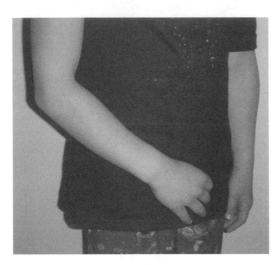

FIGURE 38.1 Nurse maid's elbow.

PROCEDURE

Two techniques will be described, both of which do not require sedatives. Both methods have equal success rates. If one method fails, the other may be attempted. Regardless of which technique is used, a "click" ensures successful reduction although it is not required. However, it has been shown that it has a positive predictive value of 90% and negative predictive value of 76%. Typically, the child is seen using the arm within 5 to 10 minutes and definitely within 30 minutes following the reduction. The practitioner may attempt a second reduction if there is no use of the extremity after the given time is allotted.

Supination Method

■ Place pressure on the radial head with the thumb of one hand and then grasp the wrist with the other hand (Figure 38.2A)
■ Fully supinate the wrist (Figure 38.2B)
■ Immediately flex the elbow completely to the ipsilateral shoulder (Figure 38.2C)

Pronation Method

■ Place pressure on the radial head with the thumb of one hand and then grasp the wrist with the other hand
■ Hyperpronate the wrist
■ Immediately flex the elbow completely to the ipsilateral shoulder

DIFFERENTIAL DIAGNOSIS

■ Fracture
■ Septic arthritis
■ Tumors
■ Osteomyelitis

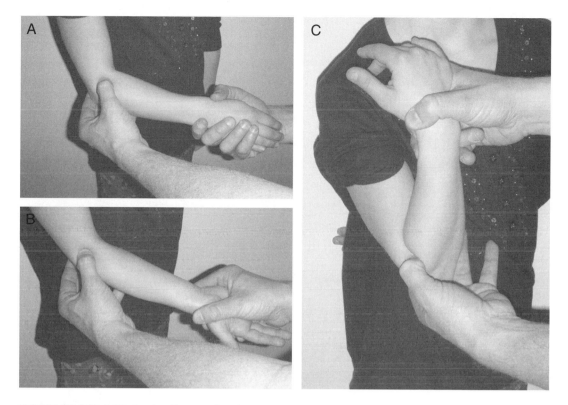

FIGURE 38.2 (A,B,C) Supination method.

Author's Pearls

- *If the first method fails, the second method can be attempted*
- *If all attempts are unsuccessful, place the patient in a posterior splint or sling, and arrange orthopedic follow-up*
- *Demonstration of the reduction on the contralateral arm may aid in decreasing the amount of anxiety for the patient and the parent*

RESOURCES

Johnson, F. C., & Okada, P. J. (2008). Reduction of common joint dislocations and subluxations. In C. King & F. Henretig (Eds.), *Textbook of pediatric emergency procedures* (pp. 962–963). Philadelphia: Lippincott Williams & Wilkins.

Meiner, E. M., Sama, A. E., Lee, D. C., Nelson, M., Katz, D. S., & Trope, A. (2004). Bilateral nursemaid's elbow. *American Journal of Emergency Medicine, 22*(6), 502–503.

Schunk, J.E. (1990). Radial head subluxation: epidemiology and treatment of 87 episodes. Annals of Emergency Medicine 19(9), 1019–1023.

Wolfram, W., & Boss, D. N. (2009). Pediatrics, nursemaid elbow. Retrieved from http://emedicine.medscape.com/article/803026-overview

39

Procedure for Splinting of Extremities

KEITH A. LAFFERTY

BACKGROUND

Splints accomplish the following: mechanical stabilization of fractures and dislocations, protection of soft tissue injury, pain control, and protection of the injured area from further trauma. Unlike formal casting, these allow swelling without the risk of external compression while giving similar short-term immobilization. Also, the patient can remove this device to perform wound care, allow range of motion, and allow continued hygiene.

PATIENT PRESENTATION

While the mainstay of splinting is for the treatment of bone fracture/injury, its use also is amenable to the following:

- Tendon pathology (laceration, tenosynovitis)
- Joint pathology (arthropathies, overlying lacerations)
- Sprains

TREATMENT

Basically splints can be made from plaster or fiberglass with concurrent use of a stockinette, webril, and gauze or an elastic roll. However, this is time consuming and for the sake of discussion, we will limit description to prefabricated splints. These contain essentially all of the aforementioned components in one apparatus. Fiberglass offers the advantage over plaster in that it is stronger, lighter, easier to apply, cures more rapidly, and does not require specific drain traps in the sink.

Proper measurement can be performed on the contraindicated extremity using an Ace wrap to approximate the length. Because most splint material releases heat as it cures, one should use cold water for application.

After proper measurement, the splint is applied and wrapped with an Ace bandage. The splint is thus contoured into the proper position and held until full hardening. When applying the splint, care should be taken to avoid the following:

- Bunching the Ace wrap
- Circumferential application of the splint around the extremity
- Tight wrapping of the Ace wrap (Figure 39.1)
- Application over a nonaddressed soft tissue wound (note that these must have appropriate wound care and dressing first)

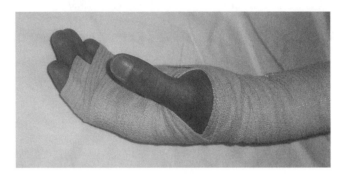

FIGURE 39.1 Inappropriately tight Ace wrap.

■ Creation of sharp edges
■ Excessive pressure points that could lead to skin ulcerations
■ Burns secondary to heat production during the curing process

The potential of a splint to induce ischemia is much less likely than that of a cylindrical cast, although it can still occur. It is imperative not to apply an Ace wrap too tightly. Also, pain out of proportion to the injury or an increase in pain should alert the provider to consider the diagnosis of compartment syndrome.

PROCEDURE PREPARATION

Unless stated otherwise, extremity position is a constant regardless of what splint is being used. In general, if a splint crosses over one of the following joints, the position of that joint should be as follows (see Table 39.1):

■ Ace wrap
■ Commercial splint roll
■ Prefabricated splint

TABLE 39.1 Positioning of Joint for Splint Application

Joint	Position
Elbow	90° flexion with forearm in neutral position, "thumbs up"
Wrist	Slight extension of 20°*
Thumb	Abducted*
MCP joints	Flexed at 60°*
PIP joints	Slightly flexed at 10–20°*
DIP joints	Slightly flexed at 5°*
Ankle	90° of dorsiflexion
Knee	Minimal flexion

DIP, distal interphalangeal; MCP, metacarpophalangeal; PIP, proximal interphalangeal.

*As if the patient is holding a bottle of beer, also known as the position of function

PROCEDURE

Upper Extremity Splints (Table 39.2)

TABLE 39.2 Type of Splint, Indication, Length, Width, and Notations—Upper Extremity

Indication	Length	Width	Note
Volar (Figure 39.2) Forearm, wrist, metacarpal fractures/ injuries	Proximal fingers to just below the elbow on anterior surface	Fully covers the forearm	Allows supination and pronation of the forearm

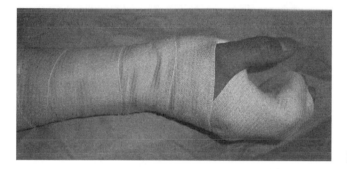

FIGURE 39.2 Volar splint.

Sugar tong (Figure 39.3) Distal radius and ulna fractures/injuries	Metacarpal heads on dorsal hand and around the elbow extending over anterior forearm to just distal to the MCP joints	Forearm width without overlap of volar and dorsal surfaces	Treatment of choice because it diminishes supination/ pronation of the forearm

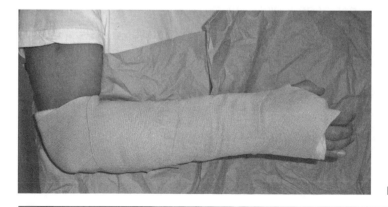

FIGURE 39.3 Sugar tong.

(Continued)

TABLE 39.2 Type of Splint, Indication, Length, Width, and Notations—Upper Extremity   (*Continued*)

Indication	Length	Width	Note
Double sugar tong Elbow and forearm fractures/injuries	Lateral proximal humerus around elbow to the medial humerus up to the inferior axilla	Fully covers the dorsal and volar upper arm without overlap	The forearm component is applied exactly as for the single sugar tong This device prevents pronation/supination of the forearm more so than does single sugar tong and posterior splint. Apply forearm portion before upper arm portion.
Long arm posterior Stable elbow and forearm fractures/injuries	Dorsal aspect of mid–upper arm under elbow along the ulna area of the forearm to the distal palmar flexor crease	Half the arm circumference	Allows some supination/pronation of forearm
Ulnar gutter Fourth/fifth metacarpal and proximal phalangeal fractures/injuries	Just beyond the fifth DIP joint to mid forearm along the ulna surface	Midline of hand on the dorsal and volar surface incorporating both the little and ring fingers	Gauze should be placed between the fourth and fifth fingers
Thumb spika First metacarpal, proximal first thumb phalangeal and scaphoid fracture/injuries de Quervain tenosynevitis	Just distal to the interphalangeal joint of the thumb to the mid-forearm along the radial surface	The width of the wrist	Splint all suspected scaphoid injuries as up to 10% of these fractures are missed upon initial presentation

TABLE 39.2 *(Continued)*

Indication	Length	Width	Note
Finger Phalanx fractures, tendon repairs/ infections, and arthropathies	No further than the joint below or above the injury	Width of finger	DIP dislocations— the joint should be splinted in slight extension or no more than 5° of flexion PIP dislocations—the joint should be at 20° of flexion
			Mallet finger is a distal extensor tendon rupture. Immobilization of only the DIP joint is required Apply splint to dorsal surface because this maintains tactile function and is in closer proximity to the bone on the surface Commercially available padded aluminum splints can easily be cut to length

DIP, distal interphalangeal; MCP, metacarpophalangeal; PIP, proximal interphalangeal.

Lower Extremity Splints (Table 39.3)

TABLE 39.3 Type of Splint, Indication, Length, Width, and Notations—Lower Extremity

Indication	Length	Width	Note
Short posterior leg (Figure 39.4) Distal tibia, fibula, ankle, and foot fractures/injuries	Posteriorly from the level of the fibula neck, around the heal to the base of the toes	Covers half the leg circumference	When this is combined with the stirrup splint, it gives increased lateral ankle support

TABLE 39.3 Type of Splint, Indication, Length, Width, and Notations—Lower Extremity
(Continued)

Indication	Length	Width	Note
Ankle stirrup Ankle sprains and minor chip fractures	From just below the fibula head running under the heal and to just below the knee on the medial surface	Half the circumference of the lower extremity	Should be able to place in a shoe for possible partial weight bearing Commercially available air casts provide similar lateral stability with improved patient comfort (Figure 39.5)
Long posterior leg Knee fractures	Posteriorly just below the buttock crease to 3 cm above the heel	Half the circumference of the leg	

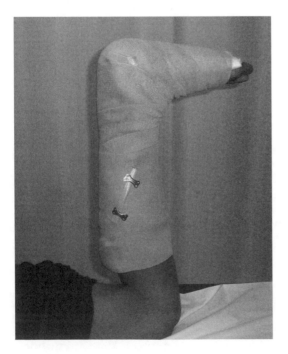

FIGURE 39.4 Short posterior leg splint.

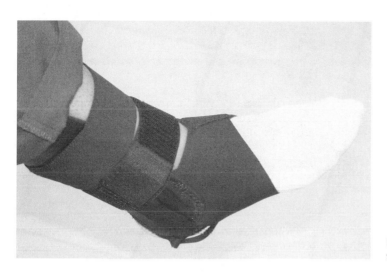

FIGURE 39.5 Ankle air cast splint.

Miscellaneous Immobilization Devices (Table 39.4)

TABLE 39.4 Commercially Manufactured Immobilization Devices

Miscellaneous Immobilization Devices	Indication	Length	Notes
Shoulder immobilizer	Proximal humerus fractures Dislocated glenohumeral joints Sprains of the shoulder	NA	Sling supports the weight of the arm, whereas the swathe immobilizes the arm against the chest wall to maximally minimize shoulder movement
Knee immobilizer	Ligamentous injuries to the knee and arthropathies	Posteriorly just below the buttock crease to 3 cm above the heel	Knee should be in almost full extension Easily removable, comfortable, and can go directly over clothing
Post-op shoe	Toe fractures/ injuries and minor foot injuries	NA	Usually combined with buddy taping of toe fractures Can be used over a splint for partial weight bearing
Buddy taping (Figure 39.6)	Finger and toe sprains, dislocations, and arthropathies	NA	Entails taping injured digit to uninjured adjacent digit Use gauze between digits to prevent maceration and/or pressure ulcers For treatment of toe fractures but not finger fractures

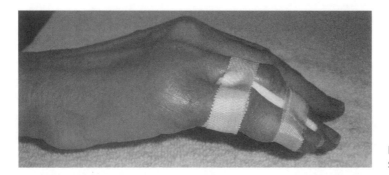

FIGURE 39.6 Buddy tape splint.

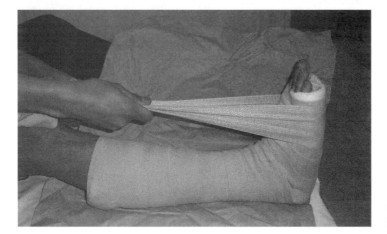

FIGURE 39.7 Short posterior leg splint patient assistance.

POSTPROCEDURAL CARE

- The importance of proper home splint care cannot be over emphasized
- Ice packs no more than 30 minutes at a time
- Elevation
- Instruct patients to return if pain increases or if there is development of numbness or parenthesis

---

Author's Pearls

- *Because occult fractures are occasionally diagnosed as contusions or sprains, splint all injured extremities: "When in doubt, splint"*
- *Increasing pain in a patient with a splint should alert the provider to consider the diagnosis of compartment syndrome or deep vein thrombosis*
- *Volar splints do not eliminate pronation/supination of the forearm as do sugar tongs. They should not be used for the treatment of ulna or radial fractures*
- *When applying a short posterior lower extremity splint, the patient can help keep the ankle at a 90° dorsiflexion by pulling up on the foot with an ace wrap (Figure 39.7)*
- *Application of lower extremity splints is made easier with the patient in the prone position*
- *Avoid prolonged periods of splint use of nonfractures in order to prevent the development of joint stiffness, which can be disabling.*
- *Buddy taping of the fingers is not indicated for finger fractures*

RESOURCES

Boyd, A. S. (2009). Splints and casts: Indications and methods. *American Family Physician, 80*(5), 491–499.

Chudnofsky, C. R., & Byers, S. E. (2004). Splinting techniques. In J. Roberts & J. Hedges (Eds.), *Clinical procedures in emergency medicine* (pp. 995–1007). Philadelphia: Saunders, Elsevier.

Gravlee, J. R. (2007). Braces and splints for musculoskeletal conditions. *American Family Physicians, 75*(3), 342–348.

Klig, J. L. (2008). Splinting procedures. In C. King & F. Henretig (Eds.), *Textbook of pediatric emergency procedures* (pp. 919–931). Philadelphia: Lippincott Williams & Wilkins.

Paras, R. D. (2000). Upper extremity fractures. *Clinics in Family Practice, 2*(3), 637–659.

40

Procedure for Managing a Thrombosed Hemorrhoid

KEITH A. LAFFERTY

BACKGROUND

Five percent of the population is inflicted with hemorrhoids. These symptoms run the spectrum from a minor annoyance with intermittent slow bleeding to extreme, excessive, and near debilitating pain.

The superior hemorrhoidal veins make up the internal hemorrhoids and drain into the portal system. The inferior hemorrhoidal veins make up the external hemorrhoids and drain into the inferior vena cava. Anatomically, the internal hemorrhoids lie above the dentate line (embryologically based, it is the delineation of anal tissue with mucus-like columnar epithelium and rectal tissue with its more skin-like squamous epithelium). Also, tissue above the dentate line (anal tissue) receives visceral innervation, whereas tissue below it (rectum) receives a rich supply of somatic innervation. Note that there is communication between these two venous systems, which form a plexus-like pattern (Figure 40.1).

Hemorrhoidal veins are very superficial as internal hemorrhoids are submucosal and external hemorrhoids are subcutaneous. Because of this, symptomatic internal hemorrhoids are beefy red, whereas external hemorrhoids are skin colored.

Internal hemorrhoids form three cushion-like protrusions at the right anterior, right posterior, and left lateral position. These normal anatomic protrusions may aid in the defecation process. External hemorrhoids form a ring-like pattern. Finally, the hemorrhoidal plexus is also composed of muscle fibers, subcutaneous tissue, and a generous arterial blood supply, which contributes to the bright red color of hemorrhoid bleeding.

Only when the hemorrhoidal plexus gets enlarged, prolapsed, or thrombosed are they referred to as hemorrhoids. Mechanistically, contributing to the development of hemorrhoids is the fact that the hemorrhoidal veins are devoid of valves and, as one ages, a loss of the surrounding support of connective tissue occurs. Further causes seem to stem from increased pressure caused from the increased venous drainage of the anal-rectum with pregnancy, portal hypertension, and conditions of increased straining (which also weaken the support of connective tissue). Symptoms are exacerbated by frequent bowel movements, prolonged sitting, heavy lifting, and any condition leading to increased draining.

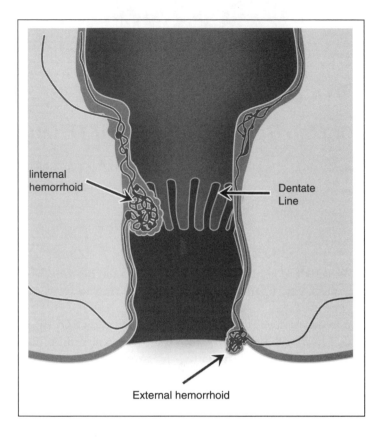

FIGURE 40.1
Hemorrhoid anatomy.

External hemorrhoids are symptomatic with either bleeding or acute pain when they are thrombosed. Internal hemorrhoids are classified according to the degree of their prolapse (Table 40.1).

DIFFERENTIAL DIAGNOSIS

- Fissures
- Fistulas
- Abscesses and other infections
- Rectal prolapse
- Gastrointestinal carcinomas

TABLE 40.1 Classification of Internal Hemorrhoids

Type	Prolapse	Reduction
First degree	None	NA
Second degree	Only with defecation	Spontaneous
Third degree	Spontaneous	With digital maneuvers
Fourth degree	Constant	Irreducible

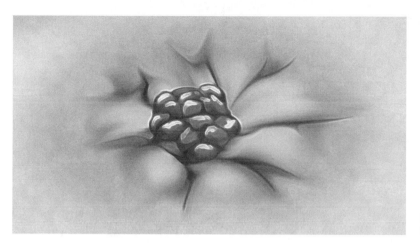

FIGURE 40.2 Internal hemorrhoids.

PATIENT PRESENTATION

Internal Hemorrhoids

- Painless, bright bleeding with defecation
- Prolapsed mucous membrane tissue (plus or minus pain depending upon if gangrenous) (Figure 40.2)
- Pruritus ani

External Hemorrhoids

- Pain (can be severe with the patient being unable to sit)
- Swelling (skin overlying firm tissue) (Figure 40.3)
- Bleeding
- Pruritus ani

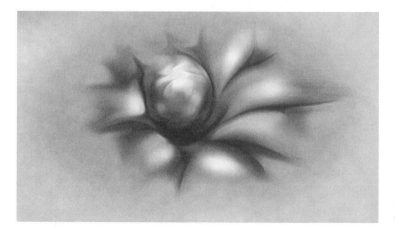

FIGURE 40.3 External thrombosed hemorrhoids.

TABLE 40.2 WASH

W	Water—increase oral intake, sitz baths
A	Analgesics—use temporarily to avoid inducing constipation. Topical anesthetic/steroid creams may be a better alternative
S	Stool softeners
H	High-fiber diets

TREATMENT

First- to third-degree internal hemorrhoids are treated conservatively with surgical follow-up for definitive treatment, which could include banding, sclerotherapy, or hemorrhoidectomy. Fourth-degree hemorrhoids require parental antibiotic and emergent hemorrhoidectomy.

External hemorrhoids that are bleeding can be treated conservatively and the patient reassured. Acute thrombosis needs to be excised—not incised. Simply incising the tissue leads to incomplete clot evacuation, reaccumulation, and persistent skin tags. It is imperative that all clots are removed after excision and unroofing of tissue. Conservative therapy consists of the acronym WASH (Table 40.2).

CONTRAINDICATIONS

- Fourth-degree gangrenous internal hemorrhoids

PROCEDURE PREPARATION

- Patient should be placed in the left lateral decubitus position
- The knee-to-chest position with the buttocks taped to the side rails is an alternative (Figure 40.4)
- Skin antiseptic solution
- Local anesthetic with epinephrine
- No. 11 blade scalpel
- Forceps
- Hemostats
- Gel-Foam
- Gauze pad

PROCEDURE

- Skin cleansing technique as described in Chapter 10
- Sterile technique
- Local infiltrated anesthesia is applied with one stick between the skin overlying the thrombosed hemorrhoid and the hemorrhoidal wall, inducing blanching that covers the entire hemorrhoid
- An elliptical excision is made in a radial manner, extending from an area just distal to the anal verge outwardly
- Unroof the elliptical excision and meticulously remove all clots with manual pressure and forceps (Figure 40.5)

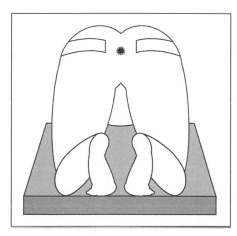

FIGURE 40.4 Knee-to-chest position.

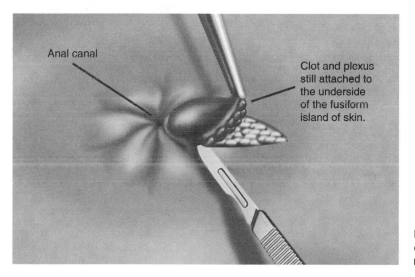

Anal canal

Clot and plexus still attached to the underside of the fusiform island of skin.

FIGURE 40.5 Elliptical excision with clot removal.

■ Place a piece of Gel-Foam in the wound and cover with a gauze pad, or place a cotton-tipped stick dipped in Monsel's solution in the wound

POSTPROCEDURE CARE

■ Conservative therapy, implementing WASH for all symptomatic discharged hemorrhoid patients
■ Note that the Gel-Foam packing usually spontaneously dislodges within 24 to 36 hours

COMPLICATIONS

■ Bleeding
■ Infection
■ Perianal skin tags

AUTHOR'S PEARLS

- *Patients get almost immediate relief of excision of thrombosed external hemorrhoids*
- *Do not incise external hemorrhoids; always excise them*
- *All that bleeds are not hemorrhoids. Although hemorrhoids might be seen, the source of bleeding could be secondary to other serious gastrointestinal disorders, especially carcinomas*
- *The painful rectal lump needs to be examined and inspected closely because the differential diagnosis is broad*
- *The prone knee-to-chest position with buttocks taped to side rails provides the best perianal exposure*
- *Bupivacaine lasts longer than lidocaine*
- *Inspection of the proximal anus and distal rectum is best done via anoscopy (Figure 40.6)*

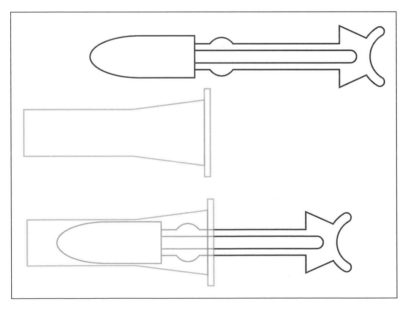

FIGURE 40.6 Anal scope.

RESOURCES

Burgess, B. E., & Bouzoukis, J. K. (2004). Anorectal disorders. In J. Tintinalli & G. D. Kelen, J. S. Stapczynski, O. J. Ma, & D. M. Cline (Eds.), *Emergency medicine: A comprehensive study guide* (pp. 539–542). New York: McGraw-Hill.

Coates, W. C. (2006). Anorectum. In J. Marx, R. Hockberger, & R. Walls (Eds.), *Rosen's emergency medicine concepts and clinical practice* (pp. 1507–1514). Philadelphia: Mosby, Elsevier.

Kaider-Person, O. (2007). Hemorrhoidal disease: A comprehensive review. *Journal of the American College of Surgeons, 204*(1), 102–117.

Nelson, H., & Cima, R. R. (2008). Common benign anal disorders. In C. M. Townsend, R. D. Beauchamp, B. M. Evers, & K. L. Mattox (Eds.), *Sabiston textbook of surgery* (18th ed.). Retrieved from http://www.mdconsult.com/das/book/body/192424659-4/0/1565/494. html#4-u1.0-B978-1-4160-3675-3..50055-1–cesec26

Sneider, E. B. (2010). Diagnosis and management of symptomatic hemorrhoids. *Surgical Clinics of North America, 90*(1), 17–32.

41

Procedure for Treating a Hair Tourniquet

LEE ANN BOYD

BACKGROUND

A hair tourniquet occurs when a hair or thread entraps an appendage; it can lead to pain, injury, and possible loss of function or loss of the appendage (Figure 41.1). Epithelialization may occur at the site of the hair or thread, impairing the ability to visualize the tourniquet. Hair has the ability to stretch when wet and contract as it dries. This tensile strength of hair causes ischemic compression as well as direct cutting action of the appendage. A hair tourniquet is typically accidental; however, incidence of intentional cases consistent with child abuse have been cited in the literature.

Hair tourniquet syndrome may involve fingers, toes, earlobes, nipples, tongue, scrotum, and penis. Most cases involve the fingers and toes, followed by external genitalia (33% of cases). Infants less than 4 months of age may be at increased risk for development of a hair tourniquet as many mothers experience postpartum hair loss several months after delivery. Our discussion regarding treatment will focus on penile hair tourniquet removal.

PATIENT PRESENTATION

- Inconsolable crying in the infant
- Painful, edematous appendage
- Presence of sharp circumferential demarcation
- Cyanosis of the appendage distal to the hair tourniquet may occur

TREATMENT

Treatment of hair tourniquet consists of removal of the hair/thread. The simplest treatment is the use of depilatory creams or the unwrapping technique. Depilatory creams are thioglycolate based, the mechanism of action of which is to break the bonds of keratin in hair. They are not effective for thread tourniquets and should not be used on open skin.

If mild to moderate edema is present, the blunt probe cutting technique may be used. The hair or thread must be visible and not too deeply constrictive in the soft tissues. If the above treatments are unsuccessful, or severe edema or epithelialization has occurred, the incisional approach may be necessary (Figure 41.2).

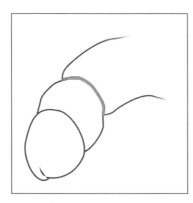

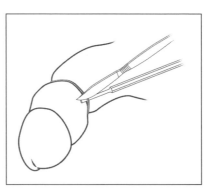

FIGURE 41.1 Hair tourniquet.

FIGURE 41.2 Blunt cut for hair tourniquet.

CONTRAINDICATIONS AND RELATIVE CONTRAINDICATIONS

■ If there is a history of an allergic reaction to depilatory creams
■ Use caution with the incisional approach in patients with bleeding diathesis

SPECIAL CONSIDERATIONS

■ All patients treated for penile hair tourniquet should follow up with an urologist within 24 to 48 hours after the tourniquet has been removed

PROCEDURE PREPARATION

Prior to initiating treatment to remove the hair tourniquet, you will need to discuss the procedure, potential complications, risks, and benefits with the patient's parents. Instruct the parents on the importance of follow-up and the expected time to return to the treatment center or primary care provider.

Unwrapping Method

■ Gloves
■ Hemostat or fine-tipped forceps

Depilatory Method

■ Gloves
■ Depilatory cream

Cutting Method

■ Gloves
■ Topical or infiltrative anesthetics
■ Chlorhexidine or povidone iodine skin cleanser
■ Fine-tipped scissors
■ Fine-tipped hemostat

■ Blunt probe
■ No. 11 scalpel blade with handle

PROCEDURE

Unwrapping Method

■ Position the patient for maximum visualization of the genitals
■ Most effective when only minimal edema is present, and hair/thread is readily identifiable
■ Put on clean gloves
■ Identify the free end of the hair/thread. If unable to isolate a free end, but a knot is present, break one end off the knot and proceed as follows
■ Grasp the free end of the hair with fine-tipped forceps or a hemostat, and unwind the hair from the appendage

Depilatory Method

■ No anesthesia is required
■ Apply depilatory cream directly to the hair being careful to avoid the urethral meatus, and allow it to sit according to the manufacturer's instructions, typically 3 to 10 minutes
■ After breakage of the hair has occurred, wash off the area with soap and water

Blunt Cutting Technique

■ Gently insert a blunt probe underneath the hair/thread, separating the tourniquet from the skin (Figure 41.2)
■ Once the thread is isolated, cut the hair/thread with fine-tipped scissors or a No. 11 scalpel blade, cutting against the surface of the probe to protect the skin
■ Proceed with removal of the remaining tourniquet material using the unwrapping method described previously

Incisional Approach

■ Universal precautions should be used at all times
■ Cleanse the skin with chlorhexidine solution or povidone iodine in a circular motion to remove debris and bacteria
■ Apply a fenestrated drape over the external genitalia
■ A dorsal nerve block is recommended. Topical anesthetics, such as EMLA cream, may be used in addition to the nerve block. For a penile nerve block, please see Chapter 6
■ Once the area is anesthetized, make a small longitudinal incision with a No. 11 scalpel blade in the inferolateral surface of the phallus at the 4 or 8 o'clock position (Figure 41.3)
■ Care should be taken to stay within the deep penile fascia located between the corpora cavernosum and spongiosum, thus preventing injury to the neurovascular bundle
■ Ensure removal of all thread/hair tourniquet

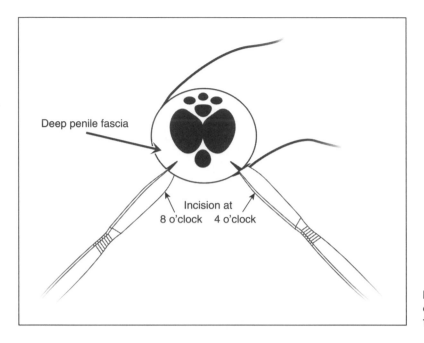

Deep penile fascia

Incision at
8 o'clock   4 o'clock

FIGURE 41.3 Incisional approach for hair tourniquet.

POSTPROCEDURE CONSIDERATIONS

- Assess neurovascular status following the procedure
- Tetanus prophylaxis if indicated
- Antibiotic therapy should be reserved for those patients who present with localized signs of infection, or those who are diabetic and immunocompromised
- Pediatric patients should be assessed for child neglect or abuse
- Urology consultation should be obtained for all tourniquets involving the penis

EDUCATIONAL POINTS

- Instruct patient/parents on signs of infection, such as redness or increased warmth of tissue, purulent discharge, or fever and to report to their health care provider
- Instruct patient/parents on signs of neurovascular compromise, such as loss of sensation, coolness to the tissue, bleeding, or dusky color to the skin distal to the sight of the injury and to report to their health care provider
- Report any difficulty eliminating urine or hematuria to the health care provider
- Instruct on importance of follow-up with health care provider

COMPLICATIONS

- Skin irritation or contact dermatitis can occur with use of depilatory creams
- With incisional method, bleeding, infection, or damage to surrounding structures can occur (i.e., urethra, corpus callosum, corpus spongiosum)
- Ischemic changes can lead to necrosis of tissue distal from the tourniquet site

Author's Pearls

- *The unwrapping techniques and depilatory creams are commonly ineffective in the clinical setting*
- *In the case of symptomatic hair tourniquet syndrome, typically the blunt cutting technique or the incisional approach is necessary*
- *Always check for hair tourniquet syndrome in an infant with inconsolable crying*

RESOURCES

Baskin, L. S., & Kogan, B. A. (2005). *Handbook of pediatric urology* (2nd ed.). Philadelphia: Lippincott, Williams, & Wilkins. pp. 2–3, 59.

Candriche, D., & Doty, C. I. (2009, May 17). Hair tourniquet removal. Retrieved from http://emedicine.medscape.com/article/1348969-overview

Procedures for Treating Phimosis and Paraphimosis

Lee Ann Boyd

PHIMOSIS

Background

Phimosis is a narrowing of the opening of the prepuce in uncircumcised patients, which prevents it from being retracted back over the glans penis (Figure 42.1). This condition may be pathologic or may be a normal physiologic finding. When evaluating a pediatric patient with a phimosis, take into account the age of the child. Phimosis is normal in newborns; by 6 months of age, 20% are retractable; and by 3 years of age, 90% are retractable. Inability to retract the foreskin in a pediatric patient requires no treatment in the absence of symptoms.

Pathologic phimosis can occur as a result of poor hygiene, diabetes mellitus, and chronic balanoposthitis. Patients may complain of edema, erythema, and pain of the prepuce with inability to retract the foreskin. Ballooning of the foreskin during voiding may occur, which can increase the risk of a urinary tract infection. Penile discharge may be present, which is often white to yellow in color, and is termed smegma, which is exfoliated skin cells. In severe cases of tight phimosis, urinary retention may occur.

Patient Presentation

- Edema and erythema of the prepuce
- Tenderness with possible induration of the prepuce
- Penile discharge—white to yellow
- Inability to retract foreskin
- Difficulty voiding in some patients with a pin-point opening on the foreskin

Treatment

No treatment is necessary for pediatric patients with asymptomatic phimosis. Treatment of mild cases of pathologic phimosis is local treatment with topical steroids as the first line of treatment. Betamesthasone 0.05% ointment applied at the tip of the penis at the area of the phimosis twice daily for 6 to 8 weeks has a 90% to 95% success rate. After 1 week of treatment, the foreskin should be gently retracted to aid in the release of the phimosis.

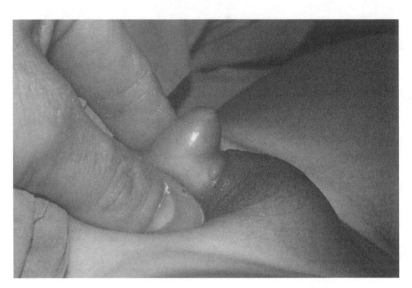

FIGURE 42.1 Phimosis.

Acute or severe cases may require a dorsal slit procedure. The foreskin is pulled taut distally and a hemostat clamp is placed at the 12 o'clock position and held in place for approximately 2 minutes, providing crushing of the tissue with resulting hemostasis; and local nerve destruction the crushed tissue is then incised. The wound edges are approximated horizontally with loose transverse absorbable sutures. The cosmetic effects of this procedure may not be aesthetically pleasing. Definitive treatment with a circumcision may be done at a later date. The dorsal slit procedure is a viable option for patients who may be at risk for general anesthesia, because it may be performed with local anesthesia.

Contraindications and Relative Contraindications

- Allergic reaction to betamethasone ointment
- Bleeding diathesis

Special Considerations

Use caution in the use of betamethasone in pediatric patients younger than 3 years. Use of topical steroids has not been studied extensively in the above age group.

Procedure Preparation

- Skin cleansing solution
- Sterile 4 × 4 gauze
- Sterile drape
- Local anesthetic (LA) (see Chapter 5)
- 5-mL syringe
- 27-Gauge needle
- Sterile gloves
- Straight hemostat

- No. 15 scalpel blade or iris scissors
- 4-0 absorbable suture
- Topical antibiotic ointment
- Petroleum gauze
- Sterile gauze
- Paper tape

Procedure

- Place the patient in supine position
- Using aseptic technique, prepare the perineal area from the suprapubic area to the scrotum using skin cleanser
- Place a sterile drape over the genital area exposing only the phallus
- Fill 5-cc syringe with LA and attach 27-gauge needle
- Anesthetize the area using local infiltration or penile block (see Chapter 6)
  - Using a hemostat, gently separate any adhesions under the foreskin
  - Pulling the dorsal foreskin taut, apply a straight hemostat at the 12 o'clock position crushing the tissue of the foreskin. The hemostat should be placed perpendicular to the corona
  - Leave hemostat in place for 2 minutes
  - Sharply incise the band of crushed tissue in between the hemostats at the 12 o'clock position using a scalpel or iris scissors
  - The wound edges should be approximated in a horizontal manner with absorbable suture using running sutures
  - Reduce foreskin to its natural position
  - Apply topical antibiotic ointment to the suture line
  - Apply petroleum gauze and cover with sterile gauze
  - Adhere with paper tape

Postprocedure Considerations

- Observe for bleeding at incision sites for 30 minutes following the procedure
- Apply bacitracin ointment to the suture line to decrease the risk of developing adhesions during the healing process
- Ensure that an analgesic prescription is given to the patient for postoperative pain

Educational Points

PHYSIOLOGIC
- Encourage good local hygiene
- Instruct on removal of smegma
- Instruct parents on gentle and gradual retraction of foreskin in the newborn

PATHOLOGIC
- Encourage good local hygiene
- Instruct the patient/parents on the importance of completing the course of topical treatment to prevent recurrence
- Instruct the patient/parents on the application of bacitracin to the glans penis twice daily for 2 weeks to prevent formation of new adhesions following dorsal slit procedure

■ For diabetic patients, encourage tight control of serum blood sugar to prevent recurrence
■ No sexual intercourse for 4 to 6 weeks postoperatively
■ Definitive treatment with circumcision may be done after acute inflammation resolves

Complications

■ If phimosis is not treated, there is an increased risk of persistent balanoposthitis, phimosis, and development of squamous cell penile carcinoma
■ Bleeding
■ Hematoma
■ Wound infection
■ Glanular adhesions
■ Tissue sloughing
■ Urinary retention

AUTHOR'S PEARLS

■ *Consider the serum glucose level and HGB A1C to rule out underlying diabetes mellitus*
■ *If the chosen technique for anesthesia is not successful, use a different technique, being cautious not to exceed the usual dosage of lidocaine*
■ *The tip of the hemostat should be palpable under the foreskin at the coronal sulcus; use care to avoid placing the hemostat within the urethra*

PARAPHIMOSIS

Paraphimosis is a tightening or constriction of the glans penis by the foreskin, which has been retracted behind the corona of the glans penis (Figure 42.2). Prolonged retraction can lead to obstruction of the lymphatics and subsequent lymphedema, which impairs the ability to replace the foreskin to its normal position over the glans penis.

Paraphimosis can occur in children, but is most often seen in uncircumcised adult or elderly men. It is often associated with poor hygiene, chronic balanoposthitis, diabetes, phimosis, chronic indwelling foley catheter, or patients who perform intermittent self-catheterization. Patients often experience penile pain and edema of the penile shaft proximal to the glans and corona, where a tight phimotic ring is present. If the constriction is severe, venous congestion of the glans is present, which can cause necrosis of the glans penis or distal urethra.

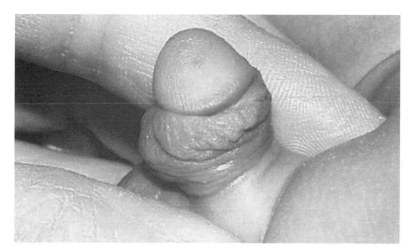

FIGURE 42.2
Paraphimosis.

Patient Presentation

- Penile pain
- Edema of the penile shaft proximal to the glans and corona
- Presence of a tight phimotic ring proximal to the corona
- Late finding of venous congestion of the glans with necrosis at the phimotic ring, which may extend to the glans penis

Treatment

Treatment of paraphimosis is closed manual reduction of the edematous glans penis If manual compression does not resolve the paraphimosis, then a dorsal slit must be performed. Consider circumcision after the inflammation has resolved. Refer to a urologist.

Contraindications and Relative Contraindications

- There are no contraindications to manual reduction of the paraphimosis
- Use caution with the dorsal slit procedure in patients with a bleeding diatheses.
- Reversal of bleeding disorders, if possible, may be indicated if impending vascular compromise is evident

Special Considerations

Careful examination should be done to rule out any area of necrosis on the phallus, which would need to be debrided.

Procedure Preparation

- Gloves
- Skin cleanser
- Ice
- 1% lidocaine gel or EMLA cream (2.5% prilocaine and 2.5% lidocaine)
- Elastic wrap or Kerlix bandage
- 25-gauge needle (optional)
- 4 × 4 gauze

Procedure

- Apply ice pack to the distal phallus for 10 to 15 minutes
- Apply topical anesthetic to the tight phimotic ring, using 1% lidocaine gel or EMLA cream
- Manually compress the edematous glans penis using gentle, steady pressure with both thumbs on the glans for 5 minutes (Figure 42.3)
- Alternatively, an elastic wrap or Kerlix bandage can be wrapped distal to proximal, from the glans to the base of the penis and kept in place for 5 minutes
- Adjunctive therapy for moderate to severe glanular edema is to make several superficial (2 to 3 mm) puncture wounds using a 25-gauge needle in the glans to promote drainage of edema fluid and/or blood from venous congestion
- Holding the penis with one hand on either side, place both thumbs on the glans for stabilization. Using the fingers of both hands, draw the foreskin down over the glans
- If the aforementioned procedure does not resolve the paraphimosis, then an emergency dorsal slit or circumcision procedure is required (see phimosis treatment section for dorsal slit procedure)

Postprocedure Considerations

- If no definitive treatment, paraphimosis is likely to occur
- Debridement of necrotic tissue is rarely indicated
- Observe for bleeding for 30 minutes following dorsal slit procedure

Educational Points

Patients and health care providers need to be instructed to replace the foreskin to its normal position over the glans penis after placement of a urinary catheter. Those patients who have a chronic indwelling foley catheter should be taught routine catheter care with gentle soap and water, stressing the importance of returning the foreskin over the glans.

Complications

- Arterial occlusion with necrosis of the glans penis
- Necrosis of the distal urethra

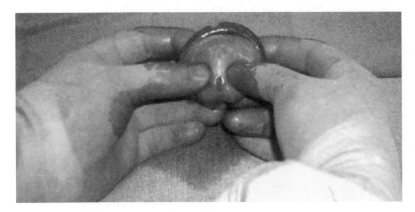

FIGURE 42.3 Manually compress the edematous glans penis.
Source: Image from eMedicine.com, 2010, with permission. Available at: http://emedicine.medscape.com/article/442883-overview

RESOURCES

Choe, J. M. (2000). Paraphimosis: Current treatment options. *American Family Physician, 62,* 2623–2626, 2628.

Ginsberg, P. C., & Harkaway, R. C. (2000). Phimosis. In L. G. Gomella (Ed.), *The 5-minute urology consult* (pp. 376–377, 388–389). Philadelphia: Lippincott, Williams, & Wilkins.

Paynter, M. (2006). Practice makes perfect: Paraphimosis. *Emergency Nurse, 14*(4), 18–20.

Pulsifer, A. (2005). Pediatric genitourinary examination: A clinician's reference. Retrieved from http://www.medscape.com/viewarticle/507161_7

Shlamovitz, G. Z., & Snyder, E. W. (2009, November 10). Dorsal slit of the foreskin: Treatment & medication. Retrieved from http://emedicine.medscape.com/article/80697-treatment

Steadman, B., & Ellsworth, P. (2006). To circ or not to circ: Indications, risks, and alternatives to circumcision in the pediatric population with phimosis. *Urologic Nursing, 26*(3), 181–194.

Tanagho, E. A., & McAnich, J. W. (2008). *Smith's general urology.* New York: McGraw Hill Co.

Suprapubic Catheter Care and Troubleshooting

LEE ANN BOYD

BACKGROUND

A suprapubic catheter is inserted into the bladder via a small incision in the abdominal wall to allow urinary drainage (Figure 43.1). A suprapubic catheter may be used for management of urinary incontinence, urinary retention, and neurogenic bladder. It may also be used temporarily after genitourinary trauma or surgery.

The benefits of a suprapubic catheter versus a urethral catheter in patients requiring chronic indwelling urinary catheters include decrease in urethral discomfort, urinary tract infections (UTIs), urethral strictures, and urethral trauma. The suprapubic catheter is the indwelling catheter of choice for those patients who remain sexually active.

Suprapubic catheter sizes may vary, but most common sizes used in adult patients are either an 18- or 20-French two-way foley catheter. Although there is no standard of care as to how often a suprapubic catheter should be changed, it is widely held that these catheters be changed every 4 to 6 weeks. More frequent intervals of suprapubic catheter changes may be necessary in the event of a UTI, or an obstructed catheter that cannot be cleared with irrigation.

PATIENT PRESENTATION

Patients may present with a variety of complaints regarding their suprapubic catheter:

- Symptomatic UTI (i.e., fever, hematuria, suprapubic pain, new onset of leakage at the stoma site)
- Bleeding from suprapubic stoma site
- Nondraining suprapubic catheter with suprapubic distention and bladder spasms with possible leakage around the catheter

TREATMENT

Urinary Tract Infection

Patients with chronic suprapubic catheters are likely to have chronic colonization of bacteria in the urine. The bacteria may consist of gram-negative organisms, gram-positive organisms, or yeast. It is recommended that patients with chronic urinary catheters not be treated with antibiotics for asymptomatic bacteriuria. However, a

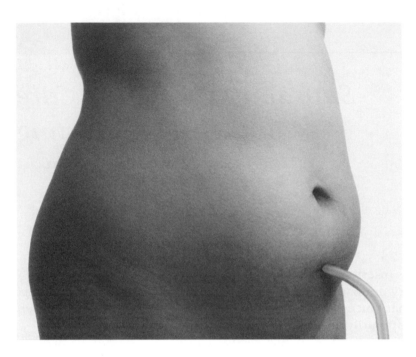

FIGURE 43.1
Suprapubic catheter.

patient who presents with fever, chills, gross hematuria, suprapubic discomfort, or new onset of leakage from the stoma site may have an acute UTI. Leukocytosis may be present. Urinalysis often reveals WBCs, RBCs, bacteria, positive nitrate, and positive leukocyte esterace.

Obtain the patient's history regarding symptoms of fever, chills, nausea, vomiting, hematuria, suprapubic pain, or flank pain. Perform a physical examination paying special attention to the abdominal, flank, and genitourinary examination. The presence of flank pain may indicate pyelonephritis or an obstructive ureteral calculus. Besides the typical findings on UA with UTI, the patient presenting with pyelonephritis may have proteinuria, WBC casts, and granular casts in patients with costovertebral angle tenderness (CVAT) on examination. Consider a renal sonogram or spiral CT scan, to rule out ureteral obstruction from urinary calculi. The suprapubic catheter should be exchanged, urine culture and sensitivity should be obtained, and the patient should be empirically treated with antibiotic therapy. In this situation, this would be considered a complicated UTI and should be treated for 7 to 10 days of antibiotic therapy. Common microorganisms associated with complicated UTIs include gram-negative organisms such as *Escherichia coli*, *Klebsiella*, *Enterococcus*, and *Pseudomonas*, with the most common gram-positive organism being *Staphylococcus aureus*. Treatment consists of oral or parenteral antibiotic therapy. Consider admission for those patients with pyelonephritis or urosepsis.

Bleeding From Suprapubic Stoma Site

Minor bright red bleeding at the suprapubic catheter site is normal for 24 to 48 hours after the initial placement of the catheter. If this is noted, do not place traction on the catheter. With well-established suprapubic catheters, the most common cause of new onset of bleeding from the stoma site is excessive growth of granulation tissue. To treat granulation tissue and bleeding at the stoma, use silver nitrate sticks to cauterize the stoma edges and the granulation tissue, being careful to avoid contact with the catheter.

Obstructed Suprapubic Catheter

Patients may present with an obstructed urinary catheter from debris, blood clots, or calcification within the catheter. Assess the patency of the drainage tubing initially to rule out kinks causing obstruction. Irrigate the catheter with sterile water until drainage is reestablished. If obstruction persists, remove the catheter and replace with the same size catheter.

CONTRAINDICATIONS AND RELATIVE CONTRAINDICATIONS

- For patients with latex allergy, use latex-free or silicone catheters when replacing urinary catheters

SPECIAL CONSIDERATIONS

If a suprapubic catheter must be changed, always question the patient regarding the date of the last catheter change. If the current catheter has been in place for more than 2 months, use caution when removing the catheter as it may be calcified. A flat-plate x-ray of the abdomen may be done to assess for calcification of the catheter prior to removal.

PROCEDURE PREPARATION

Urinary Tract Infection

- Clean gloves
- Sterile gloves
- Skin cleanser
- Foley catheter (use the same size catheter that is currently in place)
- Sterile water-soluble lubricant
- 12-cc luer lock syringe
- Sterile water
- Sterile urine specimen container

Bleeding From Suprapubic Site

- Clean gloves
- Silver nitrate sticks or electrocautery

Obstructed Suprapubic Catheter

- Clean gloves
- Sterile gloves

- 500- or 1,000-mL bottle of sterile water
- Irrigation tray with Toomey syringe
- Catheter supplies listed previously as needed

PROCEDURE

Urinary Tract Infection

- Assess the suprapubic catheter for size and patency
- A foley catheter of the same size as the catheter presently in place (to prevent difficulty in replacing the catheter in the suprapubic tract) should be readily available for immediate replacement
- Remove the suprapubic catheter by deflating the balloon, and discard in biohazard container. A corkscrew technique may be necessary to remove the suprapubic catheter
- Using aseptic technique, clean the suprapubic site with skin cleanser in a circular motion from the stoma outward
- Lubricate the catheter with sterile, water-soluble lubricant
- Place the catheter in the stoma and insert a little farther than the catheter that was just removed
- Wait for urine return. Obtain sterile urine specimen for C&S
- Fill the 5-cc catheter balloon with 10-cc sterile water (to accommodate the fluid contained in the lumen of the catheter)
- Attach the suprapubic catheter to a closed urinary drainage system
- Fluoroquinolones are first-line treatment in complicated UTIs:
  - Ciprofloxacin 500 mg orally bid for 7 to 10 days
  - Levofloxacin 500 mg orally qd for 7 to 10 days
- Patient should be admitted for urosepsis

Bleeding From Stoma Site

- Cleanse stoma site with normal saline
- Using silver nitrate sticks or elctrocautery, cauterize the stoma granulation tissue until bleeding ceases. The tissue will appear blackened in color
- Apply triple antibiotic ointment to the site and apply a light sterile gauze dressing
- Dressing should be removed after 24 hours

Obstructed Suprapubic Catheter

- Aseptic technique should be used throughout the procedure
- Ensure that there are no kinks in the tubing
- Disconnect the foley catheter from the urinary drainage bag tubing
- Using an irrigation set with a 60-mL catheter tip syringe, instill 60 mL of sterile water to irrigate the catheter
- Reassess for catheter patency. If patent, clean the distal tip of the urinary drainage bag tubing with alcohol and reconnect to gravity drainage
- If the catheter remains obstructed, replace the suprapubic catheter using the aforementioned steps

POSTPROCEDURE CONSIDERATIONS

■ Observe for hematuria following suprapubic catheter change, irrigation, or manipulation
■ Secure the catheter with tape or a catheter-securing device so that there is no tension placed on the catheter

EDUCATIONAL POINTS

■ Instruct the patient on keeping catheter drainage tube from becoming kinked, and on positioning the drainage bag below the level of the bladder to promote adequate drainage
■ Explain that minimal bleeding from the catheter is normal and may be intermittent in nature
■ The drainage bag should be emptied when one-half to two-thirds full
■ No urine output in the drainage bag and an urge to void may indicate obstruction of the catheter, and the patient should return for irrigation if needed
■ Notify the provider if fever develops
■ Instruct patient on follow-up with a urologist in a specified amount of time

COMPLICATIONS

■ Peritoneal placement of suprapubic catheter
■ Development of urinary calculi
■ Stomal stenosis
■ Gross hematuria
■ Increased risk of development of squamous cell carcinoma of the bladder

---

AUTHOR'S PEARLS

■ *Odor and discoloration may occur within the urinary drainage bag. The drainage bag may be cleaned with a solution of one part vinegar and three parts water*
■ *Patients with recurrent gross, painless hematuria should be encouraged to follow-up with a urologist for a cystoscopic examination to rule out bladder calculi or bladder tumors*
■ *Always use gentle, constant pressure; never force the catheter into the stoma*
■ *If resistance persists, use a smaller sized catheter or call the urologist*

RESOURCES

Anderson, P. J., Walsh, P. M., Louey, M. A., Meade, C., & Fairbrother, G. (2002). Comparing first and subsequent suprapubic catheter change: Complications and costs. *Urologic Nursing, 22*(5), 324–330.

Gotelli, J. M., Merryman, P., Carr, C., McElveen, L., Epperson, C., & Bynum, D. (2008). A quality improvement project to reduce the complications associated with indwelling urinary catheters. *Urologic Nursing, 28*(6), 465–467.

Gray, M., & Moore, K. N. (2009). Urinary tract infections. In *Urologic disorders: Adult and pediatric care* (pp. 92–118). St. Louis, MO: Mosby.

Shabandi, M., & Parulkar, B. G. (2001). Foley catheter problems. In L. G. Gomella (Ed.), *The 5-minute urology consult* (pp. 50–51). Philadelphia: Lippincott, Williams, & Wilkins.

Sinese, V., Hendricks, M. B., Morrison, M., & Harris, J. (2006). Clinical practice guidelines: Care of the patient with an indwelling catheter. *Urologic Nursing, 26*(1), 80–81.

Society of Urologic Nurses and Associates. (2005). Clinical Practice Guidelines: Suprapubic Catheter Replacement.

Procedure for Removal of Vaginal Foreign Body

LEE ANN BOYD

BACKGROUND

Vaginal foreign bodies are commonly seen in children and may consist of pieces of toilet tissue, fibrous material from clothing, or small toys. In adolescents and adults, broken condom remnants, pessaries, or tampons may be noted. Vaginal foreign bodies may occur as accidental, intentional during a sexual encounter, or related to sexual abuse. A child who repeatedly and purposely inserts objects into the vagina raises the concern of sexual abuse, and a sexual abuse assessment is required. Vaginal foreign bodies may also be inserted by patients as a result of a psychiatric disorder.

Vaginal foreign bodies may cause symptoms or may be asymptomatic for long periods of time. Patients presenting with symptoms may complain of vaginal discharge, vaginal bleeding, vaginal itching, odor, and, less commonly, vaginal pain or urinary discomfort. If pain is present, it may be due to vaginal distention or objects with sharp edges.

In the pediatric patient, a vaginal foreign object may not be visible on external genitalia examination. If necessary, a vaginal speculum examination will most often identify the foreign object. Further diagnostics may be indicated if observation of the object is not possible, or if extravaginal penetration of the object is suspected. Flat plate abdominal x-ray, pelvic ultrasound, CT scan, or MRI may be ordered if necessary.

PATIENT PRESENTATION

- Vaginal itching, erythema, rash, and/or edema
- Foul smelling vaginal discharge
- Bloody, brown or yellow vaginal discharge, often malodorous
- Vaginal pain
- Urinary discomfort

TREATMENT

To remove smaller objects, warm water vaginal lavage may be effective. Objects visible under vaginal speculum examination may be removed with ring forceps. In pediatric patients, a nasal speculum may be used. The foreign body may be expelled from the vagina by placing an examining finger in the rectum and applying gentle pressure on the posterior vaginal wall. Large objects may require removal under anesthesia.

SPECIAL CONSIDERATIONS

Report to Child Protective Services if sexual abuse is suspected. A sexual abuse assessment may be necessary, which includes a forensic interview and anogenital examination by a skilled child abuse healthcare provider.

PROCEDURE PREPARATION

- Vaginal or nasal speculum
  - A weighted vaginal speculum can be used for enhanced viewing
- Culturette swab
- 8 French infant feeding tube
- 60-mL syringe
- Warm sterile water
- Ring forceps (Figure 44.1)
- Nasal speculum for the pediatric patient
- Skin cleanser

PROCEDURE

- Universal precautions should be followed at all times
- Have the patient positioned in the dorsal lithotomy position for adults and adolescents, and frog leg position for infants and small children
- Ensure adequate lighting
- Examine external genitalia by holding labial traction and separation to open the hymen
- Perform vaginal speculum examination
- Small debris may be removed using an 8 French infant feeding tube placed vaginally. Fill a 60-mL syringe with warm sterile water and perform gentle lavage
- Small objects may be removed using ring forceps
- In pediatric patients, gentle compression of the vaginal wall during a rectal examination may aid in expulsion of the foreign object
- Perform vaginal culture of drainage, wet prep, and DNA probe for gonorrhea and chlamydia if secondary infection is suspected
- Swab the vagina with a betadine solution

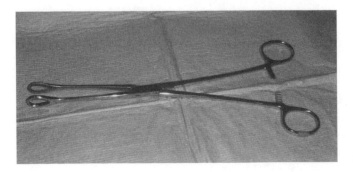

FIGURE 44.1 Ring forceps.

POSTPROCEDURE CONSIDERATIONS

■ Question the patient regarding whether the vaginal object was placed by herself or by someone else, and whether it was purposeful or accidental
■ Typically no antibiotics are necessary following removal of the foreign body

EDUCATIONAL POINTS

■ Advise the patient to return to the clinic if pain, bleeding, or fever develops
■ Discourage the use of douching
■ Instruct the patient to follow-up with their pediatrician/primary care provider in a specified amount of time

COMPLICATIONS

■ Urinary tract infection
■ Vaginal infection
■ Toxic shock syndrome
■ Vaginal fistula
■ Abdominal or pelvic abscess

AUTHOR'S PEARLS

■ *A foley catheter may be inserted vaginally alongside a foreign object to break the suction, allowing for easier and less traumatic removal of the object*
■ *To reduce the odor from a retained tampon, pierce the finger of a vinyl glove with the vaginal forceps and immediately pull the glove over the tampon once extracted*
■ *A weighted speculum can be used to enhance the view*
■ *Active or passive increases in the intra-abdominal/pelvic pressure may aid in the removal of the foreign object*

RESOURCES

Carey, R., Healy, C., & Elder, D. E. (2010). Foreign body sexual assault complicated by rectovaginal fistula. *Journal of Forensic and Legal Medicine, 17*(3), 161–163.

Kihara, M., Sato, N., Kimura, H., Kamiyama, M., Sekiya, S., & Takano, H. (2001). Magnetic resonance imaging in the evaluation of vaginal foreign bodies in a young girl. *Journal of Gynecology and Obstetrics, 265*(4), 221–222.

Neulander, E. Z., Tiktinsky, A., Romanowsky, I., & Kaneti, J. (2010). Urinary tract infection as a single presenting sign of multiple foreign bodies: Case report and review of the literature. *Journal of Pediatric and Adolescent Gynecology, 23*, e31–e33.

Stricker, T., Navratil, F., & Sennhauser, F. H. (2004). Vaginal foreign bodies. *Journal of Paediatrics and Child Health, 40*(4), 205–207.

Tolan, R. W., & Dhawan, V. K. Toxic shock syndrome. Retrieved from http://emedicine.medscape.com/article/969239-overview

Procedures for Performing
Skin Biopsy

Joseph Hong

BACKGROUND

A biopsy is performed to ascertain the pathology of the skin. Often it is done to confirm a clinical diagnosis or to help guide appropriate treatment. An old axiom in dermatology is that there are only two times when a biopsy should be obtained: (1) when you believe a biopsy is needed and (2) when you believe a biopsy is not needed. In other words, the information gained from a biopsy is almost always useful, and therefore, a biopsy is usually warranted.

To get the most information from a biopsy, certain factors should be taken into account: duration of lesion, location, healing, and interpretation. The location is important in choosing a site for biopsy of a rash or other expanding/diffuse lesion. If there is an expanding edge, this area will generally be selected, since a biopsy of the inner aspect of such a lesion will often only show necrotic cells or otherwise give an inaccurate reflection of the true pathology (Figure 45.1).

With inflammatory skin lesions, a new or recent lesion is almost always preferred. If the patient's rash is long-standing, with no lesions less than 2 weeks old, a biopsy would be of dubious benefit. A better plan would be to have the patient return when new lesions occur. A biopsy of a lesion within 48 hours of onset will give the best representative pathology and best clues for diagnosis. Evolving processes can be biopsied as long as there are newer lesions present. Of course, if malignancy is suspected, this type of biopsy can be done at any time.

Location is also important in the context of the first rule of medicine: "First do no harm." If the patient is a diabetic, a biopsy of the lower ankle will probably produce a nonhealing ulcer, which could be a more serious problem than the condition you are attempting to diagnose. Other sensitive areas are the genitalia, face, and hands. One must ask the question: Is the information to be gained worth biopsying this site? Can another site provide similar information?

Interpretation of the biopsy cannot be underrated. In this day of managed care and cost cutting, the specimen will often be sent to a predesignated laboratory, which was chosen as a cost-cutting measure. The economic realities will often be of little benefit if the specimen is read incorrectly. There are many subtleties of reading a biopsy that can be easily overlooked by someone without sufficient expertise.

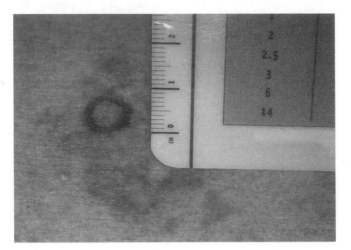

FIGURE 45.1 Lesion for biopsy.

PUNCH BIOPSY

Treatment

Generally the standard biopsy technique used for diagnostic information is the 4-mm punch biopsy. The instrument is a premanufactured cylindrical tube of stated diameter, which is used to create a hole much like an office hole puncher (hence the name). Choosing a smaller biopsy size would be appropriate for the face or other sensitive areas although 4 mm is the general size as this is enough to provide the pathologist with a good specimen for diagnosis. Another standard biopsy is the shave biopsy, performed with a straight edge razor.

Contraindications and Relative Contraindications

- Immunosuppression
- Anticoagulants (i.e., warfarin, clopidogrel)

Special Considerations

- Diabetes
- Immunosuppression

Procedure Preparation

- 4-mm punch
- Electrocautery
- Skin cleanser prep
- Lidocaine 1% or 2% without epinephrine
- Syringe
- Small gauge needle (30 gauge)
- Forceps
- Formaldehyde with specimen cup

- Pressure dressing material
- Non-absorbable suture material
- Suture kit

Suture material used is usually 4–0 for trunk and extremities, 5–0 for neck and other more delicate areas, and 6–0 for the face. A standard tray would consist of the punch, anesthetic, suture, needle driver, pick-ups, and bandage.

Procedure

Hemostasis is normally not needed for a 4-mm punch.

- Prepare the area using skin cleanser either alcohol or Betadine
- Then the designated area is anesthetized using lidocaine
  - Lidocaine with epinephrine is generally avoided for these smaller biopsies
- The punch is then applied to the skin with a single, clockwise twisting motion of the punch (Figure 45.2)
  - It is important not to reverse direction in a washing machine motion, but to keep the motion in one direction
  - This one motion will help to prevent shearing forces that can separate the layers of the skin, creating artifact that will make analysis by the pathologist much more difficult
  - It is also important to obtain a sufficient biopsy. One of the most common mistakes is to puncture only to the dermis. Generally you have to puncture through the dermis into the subcutaneous fat. This will allow the full thickness of the skin (epidermis, dermis, and the subcutaneous layer) to be evaluated. It is very important to have these layers, so that a full reading of the pathology of the skin can be obtained
- After a sufficiently deep biopsy is achieved, the specimen should be maneuvered with a needle to gently elevate the specimen above the skin and then the subcutis attachment is cut (Figure 45.3)

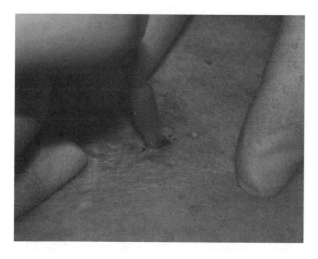

FIGURE 45.2 Performing a punch biopsy.

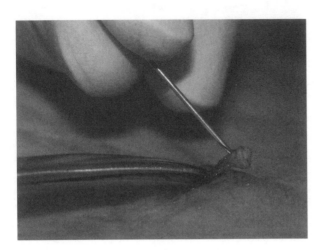

FIGURE 45.3 Maneuvering punch biopsy specimen.

- If forceps or pick-ups are used to grab the tissue, a "crush" artifact can be created, rendering the specimen uninterpretable
  - If small, single-tooth forceps are used and the tissue is handled gently, this crush artifact is generally avoided. The tissue is easier to handle this way than with a needle
- The biopsy should be immediately placed in formaldehyde for transfer to the pathology laboratory
- Once the specimen is removed, the biopsy site can be cauterized if needed, and the defect closed with appropriate sized non-absorbable suture
- Apply a bandage to the wound

Postprocedure Considerations

- Bleeding
- Pain

Educational Points

- Depending on the location, the sutures are removed after a suitable time
  - Face—5 to 7 days; scalp, neck, and arms—8 to 10 days; trunk—10 to 12 days; legs—14 days

Complications

- Bleeding
- Scarring which may lead to keloid formation

INCISIONAL BIOPSY

Treatment

This type of biopsy is used for a larger lesion, one that is suspicious of metastatic potential, or a lesion that necessitates the procurement of subcutaneous fat. This biopsy can also be called a "wedge" biopsy as it will be used to obtain a full thickness of tissue through the dermis into the subcutaneous, down to muscle.

Special Considerations

- Diabetes
- Immunosuppression

Procedure Preparation

You will need the following:

- Lidocaine 1% or 2% (with or without epinephrine)
- Suture material (nonabsorbable and absorbable; 4–0, 5–0, or 6–0)
- Pick-ups
- Scalpel (No. 11 or 15 blade)
- Skin hook
- Hemostat
- Electrocautery
- Gauze
- Duoderm or other dressing
- Sterile drape

Suture material used is usually 4–0 for trunk and extremities, 5–0 for neck and other more delicate areas, and 6–0 for the face.

Procedure

- Prepare and drape the patient
  - This biopsy should be performed under sterile conditions
- Anesthetize the surrounding skin with lidocaine alone or lidocaine with epinephrine
  - If lidocaine with epinephrine is used, wait 15- to 20-minutes before operating to allow the epinephrine to constrict blood vessels
- Ensure hemostasis by using electrocautery or heat cautery to any bleeding following the excision and then undermining under the dermal layer to allow full closure and healing
- Incise the area and then remove the necessary tissue
- Deep sutures are placed using absorbable suture through the papillary dermis. These sutures provide most of the strength and also need to be used to approximate the closure
- The skin sutures are to approximate the skin, allowing the best cosmetic result
- Nonabsorbable sutures are used; as a rule prolene or another synthetic monofilament with good antibacterial properties is used
- A subcuticular suture may be used, although the long-term cosmetic results may be inferior to other methods of closure
- Apply a bandage to the wound
- In these larger excisions that are done under sterile procedure, antibiotics are not needed, but depending on the patient and location, they may be used prophylactically

As mentioned in the previous section, the need for a proper pathologic diagnosis by a dermatopathologist is essential to provide the best evaluation and diagnosis of the biopsy.

Postprocedure Considerations

- Pain
- Bleeding
- Infection

Complications

- Bleeding
- Scarring with possible keloid formation

Author's Pearls

- *A fine, single-tooth forceps can be used in place of skin hooks with fine single-tooth forceps to help prevent stick injuries in those not used to handling or assisting with skin hooks.*

Drug Names

Generic Name	U.S. Trade Name	Canadian Trade Name
Acetaminophen	Tylenol	Panadol
Acetylsalicylic acid	Aspirin (common), Empirin	Aspirin (common)
Amoxicillin-clavulonate	Augmentin	Augmentin
Ampicillin/sulbactam	Unasyn	Unasyn
Betamethasone (oral)	Celestone	Celestone
Betamethasone acetate/ sodium phosphate inj. (IM, intra-articular, intra-lesional)	Celestone Soluspan	Celestone Soluspan
Bretylium tosylate	Bretylilol	Bretylate
Bupivacaine	Marcaine, Sensorcaine	Marcaine
Carbolic acid	Phenol (common name)	Phenol (common name)
Cephalexin	Keflex	Keflex
Chlorhexidine	Peridex	Peridex
Ciprofloxacin	Cipro	Cipro
Clindamycin	Cleocin	Cleocin
Clopidogrel	Plavix	Plavix
2-Octyl cyanoacrylate	Dermabond	Epiglu
n-Butyl cyanoacrylate	Indermil	
Dexamethasone sodium phosphate	Decadron	Decadron
Dichlorodifluoromethane/ trichloromono-fluoromethane	Flouri-methane spray	Flouri-methane spray
Dicloxacillin	Dycill, Dynapen	Dynapen
Diphenhydramine	Benadryl	Benadryl

Generic Name	U.S. Trade Name	Canadian Trade Name
Doxycycline	Vibramycin, Vibratab	Vibramycin, Vibratab
Enoxaparin	Lovenox	Lovenox
Epinephrine	Adrenaline	Adrenaline
Erythromycin opthalmic ointment	Ilotycin	Ilotycin
Ethyl chloride	Ethyl chloride spray	Ethyl chloride spray
Gentamycin opthalmic	Garamycin, Genoptic, Gentak	Gentacidin
Hydrocortisone acetate	Solu-Cortef	Solu-Cortef
Levofloxacin	Levaquin	Levaquin
Lidocaine/prilocaine	EMLA	EMLA
Meclizine	Antivert	Antivert
Mepivacaine	Carbocaine	Carbocaine
Methylprednisolone acetate	Depo-medrol	Depo-medrol (Depot inj.)
Mupirocin	Bactroban	Bactroban
Oxymetazolin	Afrin	Afrin
Phenylephrine	Neo-Synephrine	Neo-Synephrine
Phenytoin	Dilantin	Dilantin
Procaine	Allocaine	Allocaine
Proparacaine opthalmic	Alcaine	Alcaine
Propofol	Diprivan	Diprivan
Rabies immunoglobin	Rabigam, Imogam-Rabies	Imogam-Rabies
Rabies vaccine	Rabavert, Imovax-Rabies	Imovax-Rabies
Silver sulfadiazine	Silvadene, SSD	Silvadene, SSD
Tetanus toxoid	Adacel, Tdap, Dtap	Adacel, Tdap, Dtap
Tetracaine	Pontocaine	Pontocaine
Tobramycin	Tobrex	Tobrex
Triamcinolone acetonide	Kenalog, Aristocort	Kenalog, Aristocort
Triamcinolone hexacetonide	Aristospan Injection	Aristospan Injection
Trimethaprim-Sulfamafoxazole	Bactrim, Bactrim DS, Sulfatrim	Bactrim, Bactrim DS, Sulfatrim
Warfarin	Coumadin	Coumadin
Lidocaine	Xylocaine	Xylocaine
Povidone-Iodine	Betadine, Povidone	Betadine, Povidone
Benzocaine	Hurricaine	Hurricaine
Benzoylmethylecgonine	Cocaine (common)	Cocaine (common)

Generic Name	U.S. Trade Name	Canadian Trade Name
Benzoin Tincture	Benzoin, Tin-Ben	Benzoin, Tin-Ben
Polymixin B with Bacitracin	Polysporin	Polysporin
Bactroban	Mupirocin	Mupirocin
Polymyxin B/trimethoprim opthalmic	Polytrim	Polytrim
Noneugenol surgical dressing	Coe-Pak	Coe-Pak
Ferric subsulfate solution	Monsel's solution	Monsel's solution
Hydrocolloid dressing	Duoderm	Duoderm

Index

Note: Page numbers followed by "*f*" and "*t*" denote figures and tables, respectively.